Medical Terminology

Learn medical terms for nursing, healthcare professions, medical school, and MCAT

©All rights reserved 2022
MedicFluent.com

No part of this book including the audio material may be copied, reproduced, transmitted, or distributed in any form without prior written permission of the author. For permission requests, write to support@medicfluent.com.

Table of Contents

Introduction vii

Chapter 1: The Importance of Medical Terminology in Healthcare 1

    The Value of Understanding Medical Terminology 2
        1. Standardizes communication 2
        2. Eases the documentation process 2
        3. Limits errors and improves diagnostic accuracy 3
    Chapter Recap 3

Chapter 2: Learning the Medical Terms 4

    Understanding the Beginnings and Endings of Medical Terms 6
    Chapter Recap 8
    Practice Exercise 9

Chapter 3: Mastering Root Words 10

    List of External Root Words 10
    List of Internal Root Words 15
    Directional Words and Root Words 26
    Chapter Recap 28
    Practice Exercise 29

Chapter 4: Learning How to Pronounce the Medical Terms 31

    Chapter Recap 32
    Practice Exercise 33

Chapter 5: Learning Medical Prefixes and Suffixes 34

    Medical Prefixes 35
        Prefix Synonyms 37
        Prefix Antonyms 40

Direction and Position Prefixes 42
　　Measurement and Number Prefixes 43
　Medical Suffixes... 45
　　Suffixes Used for Surgical and Diagnostic Procedures.... 47
　　Suffixes Used for Pathological Conditions............... 49
　　Suffixes Used for Grammatical Function 53
　　Suffixes Used for Specialties and Specialists........... 55
　Chapter Recap 56
　Practice Exercise 57

Chapter 6: Using Medical Homonyms, Eponyms, Acronyms, Abbreviations, and Symbols. 60

　Medical Homonyms 60
　Medical Eponyms 64
　Medical Acronyms... 69
　Medical Abbreviations...................................... 72
　Medical Symbols 74
　Chapter Recap 75
　Practice Exercise 77

Chapter 7: How to Pluralize Medical Terms 78

　Chapter Recap 81
　Practice Exercise 82

Chapter 8: Understanding the Structure and Organization of the Body 83

　Medical Terms for Anatomical Planes..................... 83
　Medical Terms for Anatomical Body Positions 84
　Medical Terms for the Various Regions of the Body 86
　　Abdominal Regions...................................... 86
　　Regions of the Spinal Column 90
　　Smaller Regions of the Body............................ 92
　Medical Terms for the Body's Cavities 92
　Medical Terms That Indicate Specific Body Parts 94

Table of Contents

    Chapter Recap 95
    Practice Exercise 97

Chapter 9: Designating Root Words to Body Systems.....98
    Chapter Recap 111
    Practice Exercise 112

Chapter 10: Resources for Memorizing Medical Terms.. 113
    Latest Medical Terminology Smartphone Apps 113
    Flashcards 116
    Online Courses on Medical Terminology 117
    Guide Books and Workbooks for Reference............... 119
    Chapter Recap 120

Chapter 11: Answers To In-Chapter Questions 121

Conclusion 123

How to Download the Free Audio Files 124

About MedicFluent Team............................... 126

$6 FREE ILLUSTRATED GUIDE
PARTS OF THE BODY (SPANISH - ENGLISH)

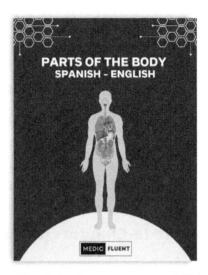

Familiarize yourself with the names of different body parts in both English and Spanish.

Inside the Body Parts Spanish-English illustrated guide, you will find:

- Illustrations of various body parts, organized into categories: the head, the body, internal organs, and male/female reproductive systems
- A table with Spanish-English translations for each body part

Scan the QR code below to claim your copy.

Visit the link below:

https://medicfluent.com/bonus/

Introduction

The world of medicine involves complex terms and a plethora of technical jargon. At first glance, these terms can seem overwhelming. This is why a basic understanding of how medical words are formed and their use within medicine becomes a vital foundation for the study of medicine.

Through this book, you will learn how to form medical terms, initially by breaking them down to their prefixes, roots, and suffixes. Additionally, you will understand that many of these medical terms are derived from Latin or Greek words, making them unique to the world of medicine.

Medical terminology also uses distinctive rules to pronounce and pluralize its terms. Also distinctive to medical terminology is its abbreviations, acronyms, and eponyms. You will understand all this and more once you have studied your way through this book.

Use this book as your resource and guide to mastering the art of medical terminology.

Let's begin with Chapter 1!

Thank you,

MedicFluent Team

PLEASE READ

- **The link to download the audio files and online flashcards is available at the end of this book. (Page 124)**
- **The answer key for each exercise is provided in chapter 11.**

Chapter 1: The Importance of Medical Terminology in Healthcare

Medical terminology describes the words and phrases used by medical professionals to understand the nuances of the human body and its functions. It is used globally to relay specific information about medical conditions and their treatments. Today, doctors and nurses are not the only ones who benefit from a basic understanding of medical terminology.

Medical billers, transcriptionists, coders, insurance agents, and even social workers benefit from an understanding of medical terminology. The terms in medicine are broken down into roots, prefixes, and suffixes. Based on how the terms are put together and used, they help eliminate possible miscommunication which might occur when using simpler terms.

Understanding medical terms make the practice of medicine seamless. Within the healthcare system, whoever treats a patient understands the precise terms to use, both for diagnosis and treatment.

From the specific parts of the body to the disease process and finally treatment, there are specific medical terms used by doctors. Based on context, doctors can sometimes use these terms interchangeably. Only those who have good comprehension of the medical terms can understand their context pertaining to a particular case.

Without the proper understanding of medical terms, it is difficult to understand specific medical conditions and their treatment protocols. It is relatively easy in these cases for confusion to arise, which can then result in the dispensing of improper treatment or medication for the patient. This is why to efficiently practice medicine a deep understanding of medical terms is crucial.

The Value of Understanding Medical Terminology

1. Standardizes communication

The main aim of medical terminology is to improve communication between healthcare professionals. Using simple terms would often limit the transfer of comprehensive and precise information about a medical case.

This is why medical terminology assists healthcare professionals as a whole. From the doctor noting down the case to the billers and insurance agents, everyone within the ecosystem can understand disease severity and possible diagnostic and treatment protocols based on standard medical terminology.

2. Eases the documentation process

When documenting cases, doctors often use specific abbreviations to describe the condition as well as possible diagnostic and treatment requirements. The simplification of these medical terminologies helps to reduce the time spent in documentation processing. This can help to increase the time available for patient care.

Another facet of standard medical terminology is that it is used globally. This means referring patients and transferring documents is relatively easy. Today with technological systems this process has become even easier, reducing the likelihood of errors and loss of documents.

3. Limits errors and improves diagnostic accuracy

A study by Johns Hopkins indicated over 250,000 people in the U.S. die annually based solely on medical errors. It is recorded as the third leading cause of death.

Without a basic understanding of medical terminology, it is relatively easy to get things mixed up which can lead to errors in the documentation process. This can result in an incorrect diagnosis or even the wrong treatment strategy. Medical terms help all healthcare professionals to understand a patient's current medical condition and past medical history.

Being able to process the information sent through the medical system accurately can reduce the annual death rate due to medical errors.

A solid understanding of medical jargon forms the basis of further studies within the field of medicine, which makes a grasp of medical terminology an asset for any healthcare professional. Along the way, it will help you communicate efficiently with both your peers and your patients.

Chapter Recap

Medical terminology forms the basis of understanding the technical jargon used in medicine. Everyone who is a part of the healthcare ecosystem, including doctors, nurses, administrative staff, billers, transcriptionists, and even social workers needs a working understanding of medical terminology. The primary benefits of medical terminology are it standardizes communication, eases the documentation process, and limits errors, improving diagnostic accuracy.

Chapter 2: Learning the Medical Terms

Medical terminology can appear to be dense and complex at first glance. For all those who are venturing into a professional field related to healthcare, understanding these terms becomes a crucial aspect of practicing medicine.

Direct memorization of the words can be overwhelming. This is primarily because of the exhaustive list of new words which the world of medicine encompasses.

To simplify the process, breaking down these terms into their key components, namely, prefixes, roots, and suffixes, is the best way to get a comprehensive understanding of medical terminology.

Prefix	Root	Suffix
Can indicate the shape, size, color or direction	Denotes the specific part of the body/ bodily function	Can denote a medical condition or procedure, or indicate the grammatical function of the word

Here are a few examples:

Listen to track 1

Transthoracic

Prefix	Root	Suffix
trans-: across (direction)	thorac-: the thorax or chest (body part)	-ic: indicates an adjective

Echocardiogram

Prefix	Root	Suffix
echo-: use of sound	cardio: heart (body part)	-gram: a type of scan (medical procedure)

Often medical terms can be generated by using a root word and suffix without the need of a prefix.

A few examples of this:

Arthritis

Root	Suffix
arth: joint (body part)	-itis: inflammation (condition)

Colectomy

Root	Suffix
col: colon (body part)	-ectomy: removal (procedure)

There are many such examples depending on what context the medical terms are used for. We will explore them in more detail in subsequent chapters.

Understanding the Beginnings and Endings of Medical Terms

There are certain prefixes and suffixes that frequently occur in medical terms. Their use changes depending on what they are describing, and it will take time for you to develop full confidence in their correct use. But understanding the general meaning of commonly used prefixes and suffixes will give you a good head start.

Here are a few of the prefixes and suffixes frequently used in medical terminology.

Listen to track 2

Prefixes/Suffixes	What they mean
Frequently used	
hyper-	excess
hypo-	less
tachy-	fast
brady-	slow
Describing size	
micro-	smaller than normal
macro-	larger than normal
megalo- / -megaly	very large
Describing location	
endo-	inside
inter-	between two or more

peri-	surrounding
trans-	across
Describing color	
chlor-	green
cyan-	blue
eryth-	red
leuk-	white
Highlighting dysfunction	
dys-	abnormal function
mal-	not optimal, ill or bad
-emia	indicating a blood condition
-itis	indicating inflammation
-osis	a non-inflammatory condition or state
-pathy	disease process
Tests and procedures	
echo-	ultrasound waves
electro-	electricity
-ectomy	removal of a part
-gram	picture or image
-graph/graphy	the procedure of taking an image
-otomy	making a cut into a part of the body
-plasty	repairing a part of the body
-scopy	internal viewing with a scope/instrument
-stomy	creating an external opening into a part of the body

Specialists and specialties	
-iatry	medical treatment
-iatrist	physician providing medical treatment
-ology	study/subject for a specific body part or function
-ologist	physician specializing in a specific body part or disease process

In essence, the root word helps to define the context of the medical term, often a body part, and suffixes and prefixes add information about a condition or disease, or a medical process related to that part of the body.

With more practice using medical jargon when speaking, you will eventually get accustomed to the terminology medical professionals use daily.

Chapter Recap

Medical terms can appear complex at first glance. To simplify your understanding of these dense terms, they can be broken down into their prefixes, root words, and suffixes. A prefix, or the beginning word, often describes the size, color, shape, or direction. The root word frequently indicates a part of the body. The root word forms the basis of understanding a medical term. Finally, the suffix, or ending of a word, indicates a medical function or procedure, or a grammatical function of the whole medical term. Most medical terms are formed using a combination of prefixes, root words, and suffixes.

Practice Exercise

Add the right prefix or suffix to the following:

1. The excessive function of the spleen: _____ splenism
   - (A) Dorso-
   - (B) Hyper-
   - (C) Hypo-
   - (D) Ventro-

2. The removal of a part of the colon: Col _____
   - (A) -ectomy
   - (B) -graphy
   - (C) -otomy
   - (D) -plasty

3. A red blood cell is a: _____ cyte
   - (A) Chlor-
   - (B) Cyano-
   - (C) Erythro-
   - (D) Leuko-

4. Indicating the inflammation of the liver.
   - (A) Hepatemia
   - (B) Hepatitis
   - (C) Hepatopathy
   - (D) Hepatosis

5. Indicating a fast heart rate.
   - (A) Bradycardia
   - (B) Hypercardia
   - (C) Hypocardia
   - (D) Tachycardia

Refer to Chapter 11 for the answers.

Chapter 3: Mastering Root Words

Root words provide the context for a medical term. Most of the root words describe a part of the body. Root words can often be divided into words that describe either an internal or external part of the body or its particular function.

For the rest of this chapter, we will look at the root words frequently used in medical terminology.

List of External Root Words

These root words are used to describe a body part or function present *on the surface of* the body.

Listen to track 3

Root Word	Meaning	Example
acr(o)-	extremity	**acro**megaly: abnormally enlarged extremities
axill(o)-	armpit	**axill**a: area under the shoulder joint covered by the upper arm
blephar(o)-	eyelid	**blepharo**spasm: involuntary closure of the eyelid
brachi(o)-	arm	**brachio**cephalic: from the arm to the head
bucc(o)-	cheek	**bucc**al mucosa: the inner lining of the cheek
canth(o)-	corner of the eyelids	**cantho**pexy: fixation or repositioning of the eyelids

Chapter 3: Mastering Root Words

capit(o)-	head	**capit**ate: largest bone in the wrist, shaped as a head
carp(o)-	wrist	meta**carp**al: beyond the carpal bones
caud(o)-	hind or inferior aspect	cranio**caud**al: direction or axis from head to tail/rear end
cephl(o)-	head or skull	hydro**cephal**us: accumulation of fluid in the head, surrounding the brain
cervic(o)-	neck or cervix	**cervic**al vertebrae: vertebral bodies of the neck/cervical region
cheil(o)-	lips	**cheil**itis: inflammation of the lips
cheir(o)/ chir(o)-	hand	**cheiro**pompholyx: itchy vesicles occurring in groups on the hands
cili(o)-	cilia, eyelash/lid	**cili**ary muscle: muscle present within the eye controlling the shape of the lens
derm/ dermat(o)-	skin	epi**derm**is: upper or outer layer of the skin
dors(o)/ dors(i)-	back or posterior aspect	**dors**al aspect of wrist: posterior aspect of the wrist
faci(o)-	face	brachio**faci**al paralysis: involvement of the face and an arm

gingiv(o)-	gums	**gingiv**itis: inflammation of the gums
gloss(o)-	tongue	**gloss**itis: swelling or inflammation of the tongue
gnath(o)-	jaw	macro**gnath**ia: enlargement of the tongue
inguin(o)-	groin	lumbo**inguin**al: pertaining to the lumbar and inguinal regions
irid(o)-	pertaining to the iris	**irido**cyclitis: inflammation of the iris and ciliary body
labi(o)-	lips or structured like lips	**labi**um: lip-like appearance, often referring to the border of the vulva
lapar(o)-	abdominal walls and flank	**laparo**tomy: surgical procedure conducted through an incision in the abdominal wall
later(o)-	side, away from the middle	uni**later**al hearing loss: inability to hear on one side
lingo/ lingu(o)-	tongue	**lingu**istics: the study of languages
mamma/ mamm(o)-	breasts	**mammo**gram: low energy x-rays used to screen the breasts
mast(o)-	breasts	**mast**ectomy: removal of one or more breasts
nas(o)-	nose	**naso**labial fold: fold of the skin between the nose and the mouth

occipit(o)-	back of the head	**occipito**frontalis: muscle stretching from the occipital bone to the frontal bone
ocul(o)-	eye	**oculo**plasty: surgery, often cosmetic, with relation to the eye
odont(o)-	teeth	orth**odont**ist: specialist managing the alignment of teeth and jaws
omphal(o)-	umbilicus	**omphalo**tomy: removal of the umbilical cord after birth
onych(o)-	nails	**onycho**phagy: compulsive biting of the nails
ophthalm(o)-	eye	**ophthal**mology: subspecialty of medicine studying the eye and its functions
optic(o)/opto-	sight	**optic** nerve: a nerve assisting with the vision of the eye
or(o)-	mouth	**or**al cavity: space occupied by the mouth
ot(o)-	ears	**ot**itis media: inflammation of the middle ear
papill(o)-	nipple	**papill**oma: benign tumor often appearing from the epithelial surface of the cell

pelv(o)/ pelv(i)-	pelvis	**pelv**ic: part of the trunk separating the abdomen from the lower extremities
phall(o)-	penis	**phallo**plasty: surgical procedure to repair or augment a penis
pil(o)-	hair	**pilo**nidal cyst: an abnormal growth in the skin which contain hair and debris, often noted at the tailbone
pod(o)-	foot/feet	**pod**iatry: a speciality of medicine dedicated to the management of disorders related to the feet
rhin(o)-	nose	**rhino**plasty: surgery to reconstruct the nose
somat(o)-	body	**somato**genic: origin from the body, pertaining to conditions or diseases
steth(o)-	upper chest	**stetho**scope: medical instrument used to listen to the internal sounds of the body
stomat(o)-	opening or mouth	**stomat**itis: inflammation or soreness of the mouth
tal(o)-	ankle	sub**tal**ar joint: joint below the ankle connecting the talus and calcaneus

tars(o)-	foot	**tars**algia: pain related to the back of the foot, particularly among those who have flat arches in the feet
thorac(o)-	chest	**thoraco**tomy: surgical procedure to enter the chest by making a opening in the ribs
trache(o)/ trachel(o)	neck or pertaining to the neckline	**trachelo**myitis: inflammation of the muscles in the neck
trich(o)-	hair	**tricho**logist: expert who examines the scalp and hair, not a medical specialty
ventr(o)/ ventri	front or anterior part of the body	**ventr**al horn: the anterior horn of the spinal cord

List of Internal Root Words

These root words are used to describe body parts or functions present *within* the body.

Listen to track 4

Root Word	Meaning	Example
acanth(o)-	thorn or spike	**acantho**ma: usually benign bump within the epidermal and squamous layers of the skin.

aer(o)-	gas	**aero**sinusitis: inflammation of the nasal sinuses observed among deep-sea divers or those who fly to high altitudes.
algesi/algia/algio-	pain	an**algesi**a: medication used to provide pain relief
andr(o)-	male/masculine	**andro**gen: steroid hormone facilitating development of male characteristics
bronch(o)/bronch(i)-	bronchus	**bronch**itis: inflammation of the bronchus, initial part of airway passage after the trachea
bronchio(l)-	bronchiole(s)	**bronchiol**itis: inflammation of the smaller airway passages found beyond the bronchus
carcin(o)-	cancer	**carcino**ma: a malignancy which develops from the cells of the body
cardi(o)-	heart	**cardio**logy: speciality in medicine which studies and deals with disorders of the heart and CVS
cellul(o)-	cell	**cellul**itis: inflammation of the skin and related tissue following infection

Chapter 3: Mastering Root Words

cerebell(o)-	cerebellum	**cerebell**ar atrophy: degradation of the cerebellum due to cancer, alcoholism or other medical conditions
cerebr(o)/ cerebr(i)-	brain	**cerebro**vascular: referring to blood vessels and flow to the brain
chol(e)-	bile	**chol**angitis: inflammation of the bile duct and related structure which allow bile to pass
cholecyst(o)-	gallbladder	**cholecyst**ectomy: surgical procedure to remove the gallbladder
chrom(o)-	color	**chrom**atogenous: production of color
col(o)-	colon	**colo**noscopy: endoscopic visualization of the colon
colp(o)-	related to the vagina	**colpo**scope: a device used to examine the vagina and cervix, primarily to detect cancerous changes
cost(o)-	rib	**costo**chondral: formed between the ribs and costal cartilage
cry(o)-	cold/freeze	**cryo**ablation: use of freezing techniques to degrade and destroy tissue

crypt(o)-	hidden	**crypt**orchidism: failure of descent of the testes into the scrotum.
cutane(o)-	skin	sub**cutane**ous: the area immediately under the skin
cyan(o)-	blue	**cyan**osis: change in the color to a bluish hue often due to an increase in deoxygenated blood
cyst(i)/ cyst(o)	vesicle or bladder	**cysto**cele: weakness in the muscle between the bladder and vagina, resulting in the bladder moving out of its position
cyt(o)-	cell	**cyto**plasm: material within the cell, enclosed by the cellular membrane
dipl(o)-	double	**diplo**pia: seeing double, or double vision
duoden(o)-	duodenum	**duoden**al atresia: absence or closure of a part of the duodenum
encephal(o)-	brain	electro**encephalo**gram: study done to evaluate the electrical activity of the brain
enter(o)-	intestine	gastro**entero**logy: speciality of medicine that focuses on the digestive system and related disorders or conditions

episi(o)-	pubic region specifically vulva	**episio**tomy: incision made in the perineum and posterior vaginal wall to aid in delivery
eryth(o)-	red	**erythro**cyte: red blood cell
esophag(o)-	esophagus	**esophag**itis: inflammation of the esophagus
fibr(o)-	fiber	**fibr**in: a fibrous protein involved in the development of a blood clot
galact(o)-	milk	**galacto**rrhea: excess production of milk
gastr(o)-	stomach	**gastr**itis: inflammation of the lining of the stomach
glyc(o)-	sugar	**glyc**emia: concentration of sugar in the blood
gynec(o)-	female	**gyneco**logy: a medical speciality involving a woman's reproductive system, function and diseases
hemat(o)-	blood	**hemato**logy: speciality of medicine studying the function and disorders of the blood
hepat(o)-	liver	**hepat**itis: inflammation of the liver tissue and related structures

heter(o)-	different, having multiple types	**hetero**genous: of nonuniform composition or character
hidr(o)-	sweat	hyper**hidro**sis: excessive sweating
hist(o)/ histio-	tissue	**histo**logy: microscopic anatomy, primarily a branch of medicine studying the structure of tissues
hom(o)/ home(o)-	identical, similar	**homo**genous: of similar composition and character
hydr(o)-	water	**hydro**cephalus: fluid accumulation in the head, surrounding the brain
hyster(o)-	uterus	**hyster**ectomy: the surgical removal of the uterus
iatr(o)-	treatment or medicine	**iatro**genic: a consequence or complication that occurs directly due to treatment conducted
jejun(o)-	jejunum	**jejuno**stomy: a external opening created into the jejunum through a surgical incision
kerat(o)-	cornea	**kerat**itis: inflammation of the cornea
laryng(o)-	larynx	**laryngo**scope: a medical instrument to investigate the larynx internally

leuk(o)-	white	**leuko**cyte: white blood cell
lip(o)-	fat	**lipo**suction: a surgical procedure to remove excess fat
lith(o)-	stone or calculi	**litho**tripsy: a non-invasive procedure used to breakdown stone, usually kidney stones
lymph(o)-	pertaining to the lymph	**lymph**edema: a notable swelling often caused due to a blockage or compromise within the lymphatic system
melan(o)-	black color	**melano**cytes: cells that produce skin pigment
men(o)-	menstruation	**meno**pause: permanent cessation of montly menstrual periods
mening(o)-	meninges	**mening**itis: inflammation of the outer protective layer of the brain, meninges
metr(o)/ metra-	uterus	**metro**rrhagia: irregular menstrual bleeding, often excessive and in between menstrual periods
my(o)-	muscle	**my**algia: pain in the muscles
myel(o)-	bone marrow or spinal cord	**myelo**blast: a immature white blood cell that is formed within the bone marrow

myring(o)-	eardrum	**myringo**tomy: surgical incision made within the eardrum, often to relieve excessive pressure
nat(o)-	birth	neo**nat**e: a newborn baby
necr(o)-	death	**necro**sis: death of cells within tissue
nephr(o)-	kidney	**nephro**logy: speciality in medicine related to the function and related disorders of the kidney
oophor(o)-	ovary	**oophor**ectomy: surgical removal of one or both of the ovaries
orchi(o)/ orchid(o)-	testes	**orchi**tis: inflammation of one or both of the testes
oss/osseo/ ossi-	bone	**ossi**fication: laying down or conversion to new bone
oste(o)-	bone	**osteo**porosis: condition resulting in the degeneration of bone
palat(o)-	palate	**palato**plasty: surgical procedure to repair or reconstruct the palate
path(o)-	disease	**patho**logy: a study of the underlying causes and processes of a disease
periton(e)-	peritoneum	**periton**itis: inflammation of the peritoneum

pharmac(o)-	drugs	**pharmaco**logy: a study of drug functions and its reactions
pharyng(o)-	pharynx	**pharyng**itis: inflammation of the back of the throat, the pharyngeal region
phleb(o)-	veins	**phleb**itis: an inflammation of the veins
phren(o)-	diaphragm	**phren**ic nerve: a mixed motor/sensory nerve which supplies the diaphragm
pleur(o)-	pleura	**pleur**al effusion: a buildup of fluid within the pleural space
pneum(o)/ pneumat(o)-	air or lungs	**pneumo**thorax: leakage of air into the space between the lungs and chest wall
poli(o)-	gray color	**poliomyelitis**: infectious disease caused by the poliovirus, which affects the gray matter of the brain and spinal cord
proct(o)-	anus or rectum	**procto**logy: speciality of medicine studying the diseases of the anus and rectum
pulmon(o)	lungs	**pulmon**ary: of relation to the lungs

Medical Terminology

pyel(o)-	pelvis or kidney	**pyelo**nephritis: inflammation of the kidneys
rect(o)-	rectum	**recto**cele: weakness in the muscles between the vagina and rectum resulting in the bulging of the rectum into the vagina
sarc(o)-	sacrum	**sacr**algia: pain observed in the region of the sacrum
salping(o)-	fallopian tube	**salping**ectomy: surgical removal of one or both of the fallopian tubes
sarc(o)-	flesh	**sarc**oidosis: abnormal inflammatory disease often of unknown origin affecting the tissues of lungs, skin, liver and lymph nodes
sept(o)-	contamination or septum	**sept**icemia: contamination of the blood often caused by a bacterial infection
splen(o)-	spleen	**splen**ectomy: surgical removal of a portion or the complete spleen
spondyl(o)-	vertebra	**spondyl**itis: an inflammation of the vertebrae
ten(o)/ tend(o)-	tendon	**tend**initis: an inflammation of one or more tendons

testicul(o)-	testicles	**testicul**ar torsion: twisting of the testicles often around its own spermatic cord
therm(o)-	heat	hypo**therm**ia: reduction in the normal body temperature below 35°C
thyro(o)-	thyroid gland	**thyro**toxicosis: presence of excessive circulating thyroid hormone
tonsili(o)-	tonsils	**tonsill**ectomy: surgical procedure to remove the tonsils
trache(o)-	trachea	**tracheo**stomy: a emergent surgical incision made in the anterior of the neck to gain access to the trachea to allow for air to pass
tympan(o)-	eardrum	**tympan**ic membrane: alternate word for the eardrum, separating the outer ear from the middle ear
ur(o)/ure-	pertaining to urine	**ure**ter: thin membranous structures transporting urine from kidneys to the urinary bladder
urin(o)-	urine	**urin**ary tract infection: infection of one or more parts that transport urine

urethr(o)-	urethra	**urethr**itis: inflammation and swelling of the urethra
vesic(o)-	bladder	**vesico**ureteral reflux: the flow of the urine back to the kidneys from the bladder
viscer(o)-	internal organs	**visce**ra: a term used to describe the internal organs within the body cavities
xanth(o)-	yellow color	**xanth**elasma: yellow fatty deposits of cholesterol under the skin
xer(o)-	dry	**xero**sis: alternate word for dry skin

Directional Words and Root Words

Directional words and root words are often used to denote a direction in which a body part faces or its position in the body. Additionally, a lot of these direction words are used in tests or procedures to inform the technician of the direction in which a test or procedure should be performed.

Listen to track 5

Root Word/ Word	Meaning	Example
anterior/ ant(e)/ ventr(o)-	in front or facing the front	**ante**cubital fossa: space in front of the elbow separating the arm and forearm

Chapter 3: Mastering Root Words

posterior/ dors(o)-	back or rear facing	**dorso**lateral: involving the dorsal and lateral aspects
superior/ supra/ crani(o)-	above or facing upwards	**supra**pubic: above the pubic bone
inferior/ caud(o)-	hind or inferior	**inferior** vena cava: blood vessel transporting deoxygenated blood from the inferior parts of the body
lateral/ later(o)-	lateral, at the side, away from the center	**latero**collis: involuntary movement of the neck from one side to the other
medial	center, in the middle	**antero**posterior x-ray: image passing from the front to the back
proximal/ proxim(o)-	close to a joint or the torso	**proximo**distal: starting from the head and torso moving outwards into the extremities
distal	away from the joint or torso	**distal** forearm: involves the wrist and initial parts of the hand
superficial	close to the surface	**superficial** vein: a vein coursing close to the surface of the body
deep	away from the surface	**deep** fascia: tissue and protective layer covering the internal muscle and structures of the body

Chapter Recap

Root words describe a body part. They are the central part of a medical term which assists with understanding the context of the whole word. Roots words are divided primarily into external, internal, and directional root words. External root words describe the outer parts of the body and their function. Internal root words describe the inner parts of the body and their function. Directional root words help to describe the position or direction of a part of the body. Directional words are also used in tests and procedures to assist in understanding how they should be conducted. A combination of root words with prefixes and suffixes form medical terms.

Practice Exercise

Complete the words with the correct root word:

1. Repair or modification of the eyelid: _____ plasty
   - (A) Blepharo-
   - (B) Cheilo-
   - (C) Hiro-
   - (D) Naso-

2. Study of the interaction of drugs within the body: _____ dynamics
   - (A) Cardio-
   - (B) Patho-
   - (C) Pharmaco-
   - (D) Uro-

3. Pooling of blood often in the appearance of a lump: _____ oma
   - (A) Hemat-
   - (B) Hepato-
   - (C) Lip-
   - (D) Osteo-

4. Yellowish discoloration of the cerebrospinal fluid: _____ chromia
   - (A) Hemo-
   - (B) Leuko-
   - (C) Pol-
   - (D) Xantho-

Choose the correct option for the following:

1. Which of the following indicates an inflammation of the bone?
   - (A) Osteoma
   - (B) Osteomalacia
   - (C) Osteomyelitis
   - (D) Osteoporosis

6. A disease or malignant process that results in the excess production of immature white blood cells.
   - (A) Anemia
   - (B) Leukemia ✓
   - (C) Poliomyelitis
   - (D) Septicemia

7. Inflammation of the digestive tract due to allergy or infection is referred to as:
   - (A) Pleurisy
   - (B) Gastroenteritis ✓
   - (C) Hepatitis
   - (D) Proctitis

Refer to Chapter 11 for the answers.

Chapter 4: Learning How to Pronounce the Medical Terms

Several medical terms have Latin or Greek origins. This can often make their pronunciations slightly complex. As with any other words in the English language, medical terms are generally pronounced in the same way they are spelled. However, some words might pose a challenge when it comes to the correct pronunciation. The letters are not always pronounced exactly the way they look. This is why understanding some basic phonology of common medical terms can help to correctly pronounce words during regular medical conversations with both colleagues and patients.

This chapter will summarize the letters which can frequently be misinterpreted in medical terms and highlight how they should be pronounced with some examples. With practice and frequent use of medical terminology, errors in pronunciation can be avoided.

Listen to track 6

Words starting with	Pronounced as	Examples
j	j	**j**aw, **j**aundice, **j**oint
sk	sk	**sk**in, **sk**eletal, **sk**ull
gy	guy	**gy**necology, **gy**necomastia
cho	ko	**cho**lesterol, **cho**ndroma
chr	kr	**chr**omosome, **chr**onic
ce / ci	si	**ce**liac, **ci**lia, **ci**metidine
ge / gi	j	**ge**station, **gi**ngiva, **gi**ardiasis

kn	n	**kn**ee, **kn**oellia
ca / cu / co	k	**Cu**shing, **ca**rcinoma
x	z	**x**erosis, **x**anthosis
psy	siy	**psy**chosis
ph	f	**ph**ysiology, **ph**enobarbital
cys	sis	**cys**tocele
cy followed by other letters	si	**cyt**oplasm
sch	sk	**sch**izoid, **sch**istosoma
pn	n	**pn**eumonia
g followed by e	j	**ge**station, **ge**nital
sc	sk	**sc**oliosis, **sc**leral
thy	thi	**thy**mine, **thy**roid
ty	ti	**ty**phoid

A few more to keep in mind		
Terms with oe or ae	e	amenorrh**oe**a, h**ae**mophilia
Addition of "thy" in the word	thi	me**thy**lene
Root word ending with g followed by a or e	j	pharyn**ge**al

Chapter Recap

It is relatively easy to confuse the pronunciation of medical terms since a lot of the words have slightly complex spellings. For the most part, the words are pronounced the same way they are in the standard English language. However, there are a few which require special attention. The continual use of medical terms will help to reduce errors over time, ensuring clear communication with your peers and patients.

Chapter 4: Learning How to Pronounce the Medical Terms

Practice Exercise

Select the correct sound for the highlighted letters:

1. **Ch**oline
   (A) ch
   (B) k
   (C) sh
   (D) si

2. **X**enograft
   (A) ci
   (B) see
   (C) x
   (D) z

3. Laryn**ge**al
   (A) ge
   (B) guh
   (C) j
   (D) ze

4. En**co**presis
   (A) k
   (B) so
   (C) sy
   (D) sk

5. **Pn**eumoconiosis
   (A) k
   (B) n
   (C) nu
   (D) pn

6. **Sc**rotum
   (A) k
   (B) sk
   (C) see
   (D) z

Refer to Chapter 11 for the answers.

Chapter 5: Learning Medical Prefixes and Suffixes

As we have observed from the previous few chapters, medical terms are best understood and pronounced when they are broken down into their prefix, root words, and suffix. For every medical word, the root word forms the context for the word.

Root words are best understood by their Latin or Greek meanings. We have just gone through a comprehensive list of root words in Chapter 3. With these root words, we will now have a look at the prefixes and suffixes that will go along with them to form a complete medical term.

Words used in medical conversation can be included in a variety of combinations of prefixes, root words, and suffixes. For instance, the word "cardiomyopathy" has two root words "cardio" and "myo" which is the heart muscle. "-pathy" is the suffix meaning a disease process. So from this medical term, we understand that a possible underlying disease process affects the heart muscle.

Similarly, a combination of root words along with suffixes and prefixes are frequently used to make medical terms. Here are the most commonly used combinations:

- prefix + root + suffix
- root + suffix
- prefix + root

This chapter will document the commonly used prefixes and suffixes that help to form a holistic understanding of medical terms.

Medical Prefixes

Prefixes in medical terminology are groups of letters or even single letters that are placed before the root word to complete the meaning. As mentioned in chapter 2, prefixes highlight the shape, size, color, or direction of the root word. Often prefixes can have synonyms, as in the case of nephro- and reno-, both of which indicate the kidney. Prefixes can also denote antonyms.

Following are detailed tables highlighting the commonly used prefixes in medical terminology.

Listen to track 7

Prefix	Meaning	Example
a-	devoid/without	**a**pathy: without feeling
an-	devoid/without	**an**esthesia: without pain
alb-	white/pale	**alb**ino: individual with a congenital lack of melanin resulting in very pale skin
auto-	self	**auto**immune disorder: a condition where the body's immune defense attacks its cells
bi-	double/twice/dual	**bi**lateral vision: sight from both eyes
co/con/com-	along with / together	**con**genital: describes a defect or deformity that is inherited genetically (i.e. it comes along with your genes)

Medical Terminology

de-	down / to get rid of	**de**hydrate: eliminate or lower total water content
dis-	separate / take apart	**dis**section: separate or open up to show the integral pieces
extra/extro-	external/ outside/ beyond	**extra**dural: outside the dura mater of the brain
hemi-	half	**hemi**plegia: paralysis affecting only half of the body
hyper-	above/ excess/ extreme	**hyper**tension: elevation in the blood pressure above the normal level
hyp(o)-	below/ underneath/ decrease	**hypo**volemia: a decrease or contraction in the total volume
idio-	singular/self/ isolated	**idio**pathic: a disease process with no known cause or occuring due to a spontaneous occurrence
intra-	inside/within	**intra**dermal: superficially given into the dermis
macro-	large	**macro**cytic: related to the large size of the cell
micro-	small	**micro**aspiration: accidental aspiration of small amounts of gastric contents into the lungs
post-	after/behind/ succeeding	**post**mortem: after death

pre-	before / in front / prior	**pre**prandial: before a meal
semi-	half	**semi**conscious: only partly aware of one's surroundings
syn-	linked/ similar/alike	**syn**dactyly: fingers that are linked together either partly or completely
trans-	through/ across	**trans**fusion: passing blood or blood products through an intravenous route
ultra-	extreme / out of the normal	**ultra**sound: sound waves traveling at a high-frequency

Prefix Synonyms

As briefly mentioned earlier in this chapter, a few prefixes have more than one variety. This is primarily since a lot of words used to form medical terms are sourced from Latin and Greek, which has resulted in some terms having prefixes from both languages. In many instances, only one or the other is used based on the context of the word being formed. However, in certain cases, more than one type of prefix can be used.

The next section will highlight all the synonymous prefixes.

Body parts with more than one prefix

Listen to track 8

Body Part	Greek Prefix	Latin Prefix
Breast	mast(o)- **mast**itis: inflammation of the breast tissue	mamm(o)- **mammo**plasty: surgical procedure to repair or augment the breasts
Kidneys	nephr(o)- **nephro**logy: medical specialty studying the function of the kidneys and related diseases	ren(o)- **ren**al calculi: kidney stones
Navel	omphal(o)- **omphal**itis: infection of the umbilical stump resulting in inflammation	umbilic(o)- **umbilico**plasty: surgical repair or augmentation of the umbilicus
Teeth	odont(o)- **odont**oma: benign tumor related to the development of the teeth	dent(o)- **dent**ist: specialist who studies and treats conditions related to the teeth

Additional Synonymous Prefixes

Listen to track 9

Word meaning	Prefix synonyms	Examples
faulty/difficult/painful	dys-	**dys**phagia: a difficulty swallowing
	mal-	**mal**formation: a body part that has not been formed correctly or completely
against	anti-	**anti**dote: a substance or drug used to counteract another toxic substance
	contra-	**contra**indication: not indicated to be taken on used in certain situations
both/dual	ambi-	**ambi**dextrous: the ability to use both the right and left hand equally
	bi-	**bi**cuspid: consisting of dual cusps or leaflets, as seen with heart valve
	di-	**di**gastric muscle: jaw muscle which has two bellies

above	epi-	**epi**dermis: the uppermost layer of the skin
	super-	**super**ciliary: prominence noted above the eyes, the eyebrow
	supra-	**supra**clavicular: the area above the clavicles, in the upper neck region
under	hypo-	**hypo**tonia: a decrease in the muscle tone
	infra-	**infra**patellar: below the knee
	sub-	**sub**ungual: beneath the nails

Prefix Antonyms

Identifying the prefixes of a medical term assists with understanding the whole term. While a lot of the prefixes help with directly assigning a meaning to the root word, a few prefixes are used to indicate opposite meanings to specific root words. These antonyms can come in pairs where each one refers to the opposite form of the root word. The following chart highlights the prefix antonyms used in medical terminology.

Listen to track 10

Prefix	Meaning	Example
ab-	move away from	**ab**ductor: muscle or force moving away from the median

ad-	move toward	**ad**ductor: muscle or force favoring the movement toward the median
bio-	life	**bio**logy: the study of life and living things
necro-	death	**necro**sis: process of decay or death of the cells and tissues
brady-	slow	**brady**cardia: slowing down of the heart rate
tachy-	fast	**tachy**pnea: rapid breathing rate
endo-	in/within	**endo**genous: formed or sourced from inside or within the body
exo-	out/exterior	**exo**crine glands: those that facilitate secretions onto the surface of the skin
eu-	normal/ regular	**eu**thyroid: normal state of the thyroid gland and hormone production
dys-	irregular function / not well	**dys**plasia: abnormal cells within a particular tissue sample
hyper-	excess / more than	**hyper**tonia: excessive muscle tone
hypo-	little/ less than	**hypo**plasia: incomplete development due to an insufficient number of cells

antero-	forward	**antero**grade amnesia: inability to form new memories after a traumatic incident on the brain
retro-	backward	**retro**grade flow: the flow of the body fluid is in the backward or opposite direction

Direction and Position Prefixes

Listen to track 11

Prefix	Meaning	Example
circum-	around	**circum**cision: surgical procedure to remove the foreskin surrounding the tip of the penis
dia-	through	**dia**lysis: often done to facilitate kidney function by removing toxins in the blood through an external machine
in-	inside	**in**tubation: procedure to insert a tube into a body cavity
inter-	between	**inter**articular: between two surfaces of a joint
intra-	within	**intra**venous: within the veins, or inserting into the veins

juxta-	alongside / next to	**juxta**glomerular: situated next to the glomerulus in the kidneys
meso-	middle	**meso**derm: middle of the three layers of the germ cells
opisth(o)-	back/behind/rear	**opisth**otic: bony elements situated behind the inner ear
para-	next to / adjacent to	**para**vertebral: next to or beside the length of the vertebrae
peri-	around	**peri**umbilical: around the umbilical area
pre-	before	**pre**operative: before a surgical process
pro-	in front of	**pro**gnosis: estimating the outcome of a condition or situation based on facts collected beforehand
re-	again/back	**re**lapse: movement to a previous situation or condition

Measurement and Number Prefixes

We have seen a few prefixes which denote either a greater-than or lesser-than state. Two such prefixes are **hypo-** and **hyper-**, which suggest something is either more than or less than its normal capacity. Examples include hypotonia or hypertonia, indicating an increase or decrease in muscle tone.

However, these prefixes designate subjective amounts and not a specific quantity. The following table will highlight a few prefixes that specifically indicate quantities and are frequently used to form medical terms.

Listen to track 12

Prefix	Meaning	Example
deci-	one-tenth	**deci**bel: measuring one-tenth of a bel, measuring the loudness of sound
kilo-	1,000	**kilo**gram: denoting a thousand grams
milli-	one thousandth	**milli**meter: one-thousandth of a meter
mono-	one	**mono**neuropathy: disease or injury to a single nerve
nulli-	zero	**nulli**para: a woman who has never had children
primi-	first	**primi**para: a woman who has given birth for the first time
quadri-	four	**quadri**ceps femoris: largest muscle group in the thigh which is divided into four distinct sections within the thigh
semi-	half	**semi**conscious: partially conscious
tetra-	four	**tetra**plegia: paralysis of the upper limbs and lower limbs

tri-	three	**tric**eps: muscle present in the dorsal aspect of the upper arm, consisting of three distinct parts: long, medial and lateral heads
uni-	one	**uni**lateral: only on one side

Medical Suffixes

Suffixes are added to the ending of a medical term to indicate either a medical condition or procedure. In some cases, they help to modify the grammatical function of the word. Often several suffixes have similar meanings, such as -osis and -pathy, both of which highlight disease processes; however, the suffix used will change based on the root word used.

The following f tables list the most commonly used suffixes in medical terminology.

Listen to track 13

Suffix	Meaning	Example
-cyte	cell	leuko**cyte**: white blood cell
-cytosis	referring to a cell and its particular functions	phago**cytosis**: a cell whose primary function is to eat (phago) microorganisms, dead cells, and foreign particles
-esis	condition/disease process/symptom	encopr**esis**: fecal incontinence

-spasm	involuntary muscle contraction	broncho**spasm**: smooth muscle contraction resulting in constriction of the bronchus
-stasis	stagnant / remaining at the same level	hemo**stasis**: repair process that results in the slowing down of bleeding through a vessel following injury
-stenosis	narrowing/closure of a passage	aorto**stenosis**: narrowing of the aorta either due to a disease process or congenital malformation
-tion	referring to either a process or state	inges**tion**: a process of taking in food or drink
-toxic	harmful/ poisonous	cyto**toxic**: harmful to the living cells of the body
-uria	refers to the passage of urine, often a related abnormality	dys**uria**: difficulty or pain with passing urine
-y	state or condition, can be a normal or abnormal process	dactyl**y**: the normal arrangement of fingers and toes

Suffixes Used for Surgical and Diagnostic Procedures

Listen to track 14

Suffix	Meaning	Example
-centesis	a procedure conducted for the removal of fluid from a space or cavity	arthro**centesis**: removal of synovial fluid from a joint space
-clasis	action of crushing	osteo**clasis**: intentional fractures made in the bone by a surgeon for corrective realignment
-desis	procedure to bind or fuse surfaces	pleuro**desis**: procedure to reduce the area between the chest and lungs to prevent the accumulation of either fluid or air
-ectomy	surgical procedure to remove a part of an organ or collect tissue	gast**rectomy**: procedure to either partially or completely remove a part of the stomach
-gram	the procedure of recording or using equipment such as an X-ray for a test	encephalo**gram**: procedure to record the electrical activity of the brain is
-graph	tool used to record results from a procedure	cardio**graph**: a device which displays the electrical activity of the heart for further analysis

-graphy	procedure wherein CT or X-ray images are produced	angio**graphy**: procedure which uses radio-opaque substances to visualize the structure and flow within blood vessels and lymph using CT or X-rays
-meter	device used to record specific measurements	sphygmomano**meter**: device used to measure the blood pressure
-metry	process of obtaining measurements	spiro**metry**: study done to measure the lung capacity during different physical states
-opsy	checking or examining	bi**opsy**: examination of a sample tissue taken from the body
-pexy	surgical procedure aimed to repair	orchio**pexy**: surgical procedure which moves an undescended testicle into the scrotum
-plasty	reconstructive surgical procedure	angio**plasty**: repair of a blocked or narrowed blood vessel
-rrhaphy	closing exposed surfaces or wounds with sutures	neuro**rrhaphy**: surgically suturing nerves that have been divided

-scope	instrument used to internally visualize a cavity or particular organ	procto**scope**: device used to internally visualize the anus and external parts of the rectum
-scopy	procedure involving the internal visualization a cavity or particular organ	endo**scopy**: internal visualization of the GI tract using a flexible tube
-stomy	procedure to make an external opening into the body	colo**stomy**: procedure to create an external opening in the large colon
-tomy	procedure to cut and gain access into a cavity	laparo**tomy**: incision created in the abdomen to gain access into the abdominal cavity

Suffixes Used for Pathological Conditions

Listen to track 15

Suffix	Meaning	Example
-algia	pain	my**algia**: muscle pain
-asthenia	reduction in strength/ capacity	my**asthenia** gravis: autoimmune disorder resulting in the reduction of neuromuscular strength especially of the voluntary muscles

-cele	herniation or protrusion of a body part	recto**cele**: weakness in the muscles surrounding the rectum resulting in herniation into the vagina
-dynia	pain	neuro**dynia**: pain in a region of the specific nerves
-ectasia/ ectasis	dilation within a hollow organ	telangi**ectasia**: widening of the blood vessels, especially those closer to the surface of skin or mucous membranes
-edema	accumulation of excess fluids within tissues or body cavities	lymph**edema**: accumulation of fluid, specifically lymph, within the lymphatic system
-emesis	vomiting	hemat**emesis**: the vomiting of blood
-emia	blood condition	septic**emia**: infection of the blood
-ia	specific condition	insomn**ia**: psychological or physical condition resulting in an inability to sleep
-iasis	abnormal state	mydr**iasis**: pupils that are dilated often beyond a normal state
-ism	condition of specific part of the body	priap**ism**: painful erection of the penis

-itis	inflammation	arth**itis**: inflammation of the joints
-lith	stone/calculus	oto**lith**: mineralized crystals within the inner ear which assist with hearing
-lysis	breakdown	auto**lysis**: self-digestion of cells by their own enzymes, often noted with damaged or dead cells
-lytic	decomposition/ inhibition	osteo**lytic**: dissolution or punched out areas within bones
-megaly	abnormal enlargement	cardio**megaly**: abnormal enlargement of the heart
-malacia	soften/weaken	osteo**malacia**: weakening of the bones
-oma/ma	malignancy/ tumor	oste**oma**: growth of bone, usually on another bony surface
-osis	abnormal condition or state	thromb**osis**: condition where excessive clots are formed within the blood, blocking blood vessels
-pathy	dysfunction or disease process	neuro**pathy**: disease resulting in dysfunction of one or more nerves
-penia	lack of	thrombocyto**penia**: decrease in level of platelets

-phobia	increased sensitivity or fear of	photo**phobia**: increased sensitivity to light
-plegia	paralysis	hemi**plegia**: paralysis noted only on one side of the body
-ptosis	downward displacement or drooping	uvulo**ptosis**: falling of the palate, usually after relaxation and elongation
-rrhage/ rrhagia	abnormally excessive flow, often following a rupture	meno**rrhagia**: excessive blood flow during menses
-rrhea	excessive flow or discharge	dia**rrhea**: passage of excessive loose and watery stools
-rrhexis	rupture of organ or vessel	angio**rrhexis**: rupture of blood vessels
-sclerosis	hardening	oto**sclerosis**: irregular bone growth or hardening of the middle ear bones

Suffixes Used for Grammatical Function

Listen to track 16

Suffix	Example
Suffixes used as an adjective to describe an organ, disease process, or condition:	
-ac	celi**ac**: affecting or part of the abdomen
-al	rect**al**: pertaining to the rectum
-ar	ventricul**ar**: connected to is a part of the ventricle
-ary	coron**ary**: related to the coronary blood vessels
-eal	esophag**eal**: related to the esophagus
-ic	gastr**ic**: pertaining to the stomach
-oid	muc**oid**: resembles mucus
-ous	eczemat**ous**: related to or can cause eczema
-tic	caus**tic**: corrosive or can burn living tissue
Suffixes used to change a noun to a verb:	
-ate	coagul**ate**: solidify or congeal, especially within blood vessels
	hydr**ate**: infuse or take up water
-ize	cauter**ize**: cause burns on flesh either with an instrument or a substance

A few suffixes can have more than one grammatical function:

-genic caused by / causing / related to a gene	hemato**genic**: related to or caused by blood fibrino**genic**: resulting in the development of fibers trans**genic**: process to alter genes of a living organism
-ory characteristics/ ability/organ	sens**ory**: used for feeling or perception circulat**ory**: referring to the system used to transport blood to and from the heart
-ile characteristics/ ability/condition	erect**ile**: ability to become erect febr**ile**: fever or raise in temperature

Suffixes used to indicate the singular forms of nouns:

-um	cerebell**um**: present on the inferior and posterior part of the brain just above the spinal cord
-us	Enterococc**us**: singular form of the gut bacteria

Suffixes used to scale down size:

-icle	vesi**cle**: small fluid-filled sac
-ole	bronchi**ole**: smallest branch of the respiratory system
-ula	mac**ula**: non-elevated pigmented skin patches
-ule	nod**ule**: growth or lump, can be malignant

Suffixes Used for Specialties and Specialists

Listen to track 17

Suffix	Meaning	Example
-iatry	particular field of medicine	psych**iatry**: medical study and diagnosis of mental health conditions
-ician	professional belonging to a specific field of study	pediat**rician**: medical expert in the field pediatrics which involves child health and wellness
-ist	certified practitioner	biolog**ist**: an expert who studies or researches on living organisms
-ology	study	cardi**ology**: the study of the heart and related functions and conditions
-ologist	professional belonging to a specific field of study	nephr**ologist**: specialist who studies and diagnoses conditions relating to the kidneys and urinary system
-trics	medicine/doctor/treatment	obste**trics**: field of medicine dealing with pregnancy, birth and the postpartum phase

Chapter Recap

Medical terms are made up of prefixes, root words, and suffixes. Medical prefixes and suffixes are used to further describe root words. Different combinations of prefixes, root words, and suffixes can be used to form complete medical terms.

Medical prefixes form the beginning of medical terms. They are used to describe a direction, shape, color, or size. Some prefixes can be synonymous based on the context they are being used for. Synonymous prefixes can also exist if their origin is from either the Greek or Latin script (especially for organs). Some prefixes are used as antonyms for the root word, where they depict opposite meanings for the root word.

Medical suffixes are used to form the ending of a medical term. It is used to describe a medical process or condition. In some instances, suffixes have a grammatical function to provide context to the rest of the medical term. Some suffixes can be used for more than one function. Additionally, suffixes can denote a medical specialty or specialist or describe a type of medical procedure.

Practice Exercise

Select the correct option for the highlighted prefix or suffix:

1. Arthro**desis**
   (A) Disease process
   (B) Fusion of two surfaces
   (C) Removal of fluid
   (D) Removal of organ part

2. **Hemi**hypertrophy
   (A) One
   (B) Complete
   (C) Four
   (D) Half

3. **Mal**rotation
   (A) Against
   (B) Above
   (C) Dual
   (D) Faulty

4. Phlebo**tomy**
   (A) Creation of an external opening
   (B) Procedure to internally visualize organs
   (C) Procedure to gain access into a cavity
   (D) Surgical reconstruction

5. **Intra**mural
   (A) Around
   (B) Between
   (C) Beyond
   (D) Within

Refer to Chapter 11 for the answers.

Chapter "Good Will"

Helping others without expectation of anything in return has been proven to lead to increased happiness and satisfaction in life.

We would love to give you the chance to experience that same feeling during your reading or listening experience today...

All it takes is a few moments of your time to answer one simple question:

<u>Would you make a difference in the life of someone you've never met—without spending any money or seeking recognition for your good will?</u>

If so, we have a small request for you.

If you've found value in your reading or listening experience today, we humbly ask that you take a brief moment right now to leave an honest review of this book. It won't cost you anything but 30 seconds of your time—just a few seconds to share your thoughts with others.

Your voice can go a long way in helping someone else find the same inspiration and knowledge that you have.

Scan the QR code below:

OR

Visit the link below:

https://geni.us/9bEwEM

Thank you in advance!

Chapter 6: Using Medical Homonyms, Eponyms, Acronyms, Abbreviations, and Symbols

Medical Homonyms

Homonyms refer to words that are pronounced similarly but have spellings and meanings that are different.

An example of this is "humorous" and "humerus." The first refers to something funny or having the capability of being funny, whereas the second is a medical term referring to the long bone in the forearm. With this example, it is easier to understand which word is intended from the different contexts the words are used in. However, with two similar sounding medical terms, it might not be so easy.

This makes it important to clarify doubts when they arise. Especially in medical conversations when words are used without knowing the actual spelling of the word.

We will now take a look at the most frequently used medical homonyms.

Listen to track 18

Agonist	Antagonist
a chemical that activates a receptor to produce a biological response	a chemical that blocks the action of an agonist on a receptor
Anuresis	**Enuresis**
an inability to pass urine	urinary incontinence, frequently observed while sleeping

Apophysis	Epiphysis
a natural protuberance from the bone	the distal end of the long bone which grows and then finally ossifies separately from the shaft
Aural	**Oral**
related to the ear or its functions	related to the mouth or its functions; can also refer to a direction conveyed by speaking
Diathesis	**Diastasis**
predisposition to a state or condition, especially when considering disease	condition where a fused body part, either a bone or muscle, separates
Dyskaryosis	**Dyskeratosis**
cytological changes observed in the squamous epithelial changes, noted by hyperchromatic nuclei containing irregular nuclear chromatin	abnormal and often increased keratinization noted below the stratum granulosum, which results in hardening of skin, hair or nails
Dysphagia	**Dysphasia**
difficulty or painful swallowing	decrease in the ability to comprehend and form cohesive speech
Galactorrhea	**Galacturia**
an abnormal increase in the flow of milk from the breasts	milky appearance of the urine

Humeral	**Humoral**
related to the humerus	related to the body fluids
Ileum	**Illium**
Third section of the small colon, after the jejunum and before cecum of the large colon	large broad bone forming the upper portion of the pelvic bone
Lice	**Lyse**
parasites which affect the hair-bearing parts of the body, primarily the head and pubis	breakdown or destroy
Malleolus	**Malleus**
bony projection in the ankle shaped like a hammer head or mallet	first ossicle in the middle ear, shaped like a hammer
Mucous	**Mucus**
adjective; meaning the production of mucus from mucous-membranes	noun; meaning the sticky fluid which acts as a lubricant and protects internal layers
Osteal	**Ostial**
resembles or is related to the bone or its functions	related to the os/ostium which is an opening
Profuse	**Perfuse**
excessive flow, often referred for the excessive flow of blood	supplying a tissue or organ with fluid

Chapter 6: Using Medical Homonyms, Eponyms, Acronyms, Abbreviations, and Symbols

Radicle	**Radical**
smallest division, root, often the beginning of a blood vessel or nerve	extreme measures taken to bring about a change especially when dealing with difficult to treat conditions such as cancer
Resection	**Recession**
surgical removal of a specific part or organ	corrective procedure for strabismus *alternate meaning* a movement away from its normal position, such as the hairline or gum line
Tract	**Track**
anatomical passage formed by the organization of organs within the system, such as the gastrointestinal tract *alternate meaning* abnormal passage formed as a result of a disease process e.g., fistula	refers to a route, often for administration
Vesical	**Vesicle**
reference to the urinary bladder	small fluid-filled sac; can be a normal anatomical structure or related to an abnormal disease process
Viscous	**Viscus**
used to describe a fluid consistency which is sticky and thick	an internal organ of the body

Medical Eponyms

Eponyms are simply terms in the language that comes from the proper name of a person or place. Derived from the Greek word *eponymous*, which means "given as a name," eponyms help to make some portion of the medical language unique and also assist with designating specific procedures, physical signs, or even anatomical parts.

Following is a list of the most frequently used eponyms in medical language.

Listen to track 19

Eponym	Meaning	Eponym Reference
Achilles tendon	This tendon is located in the back of the leg connecting the muscles in the leg to the calcaneus or heel bone.	Reference to the Greek warrior Achilles, who was especially vulnerable on his heel.
Addison's disease	A disease characterized by a loss of adrenal hormones such as cortisol and aldosterone, due to a disease process resulting in adrenal insufficiency.	Named after Dr. Thomas Addison who discovered this group of symptoms displaying characteristic findings in the 1950s.

Chapter 6: Using Medical Homonyms, Eponyms, Acronyms, Abbreviations, and Symbols

Allis clamp	A surgical clamp that assists in holding soft tissues during procedures.	Oscar Huntington Allis introduced this instrument in the 1880s.
Alzheimer's disease	Progressive brain atrophy which results in the loss of basic mental faculties, such as memory and cognition.	Named after German psychiatrist Alois Alzheimer who identified his first case in 1901.
Apgar score	A quick score formulated on specific criteria to determine the health of a neonate shortly after birth.	Developed in 1952 by anesthesiologist Virginia Apgar as a standardized way to evaluate infants at birth.
Bartholin's glands	Small glands located on either side of the vaginal opening which assist in lubrication by secreting mucus.	Caspar Bartholin II discovered these glands in the 17th century.
Bell's palsy	A paralysis of the facial nerve which results in a decrease in the function of the muscles innervated by the nerve.	Neurophysiologist Sir Charles Bell detailed the anatomical changes from idiopathic facial nerve paralysis.

Broca's aphasia	Injury to the ventroposterior portions of the brain resulting in an inability to form words.	Named after French neurologist Paul Broca.
Cushing's syndrome	A collection of symptoms, which include weight gain, collection of fat in the neck and shoulders, and abnormal hair growth, due to exposure to elevated levels of cortisol.	Harvey William Cushing described Cushing's Syndrome/Disease in 1932. Cushing's reflex is also named after him, a brain reaction due to compression.
Down syndrome	A collection of features and symptoms such as a flattened nose, mental retardation, and short stature among those who have trisomy 21.	John Langdon Down described the features of Down's syndrome in 1862.
Eustachian tube	An auditory tube that connects the middle ear to the nasopharynx. Its primary function is to equalize pressure.	This tube is named after anatomist Bartolomeo Eustachi.

Chapter 6: Using Medical Homonyms, Eponyms, Acronyms, Abbreviations, and Symbols

Friedreich's ataxia	This is an autosomal recessive motor neuron genetic disorder that affects the ability to walk, along with a loss of sensation in the arms and legs.	This genetic condition is named after the German pathologist and neurologist Nikolaus Friedreich.
Grey Turner's sign	Bruising and bluish discoloration of the flanks, indicating retroperitoneal hemorrhage. This is used as a sign to indicate acute pancreatitis.	The sign is named after the British surgeon George Grey Turner.
Heimlich maneuver	This is an emergency maneuver conducted when someone is choking. Abdominal thrusts are performed to eliminate the foreign body from the respiratory pathway.	This maneuver is named after American thoracic surgeon Henry Judah Heimlich.

Hodgkin lymphoma	Excessive proliferation of a specific type of lymphocyte is observed with Hodgkin lymphoma. Fever, night sweats, weight loss, and enlarged lymph nodes are symptoms observed.	Described in 1832 by British pathologist Thomas Hodgkin.
Homans' sign	Discomfort observed behind the knee following forced dorsiflexion of the foot. Used as a sign to indicate deep vein thrombosis.	In 1941 American surgeon John Homans consistently observed this positive sign in patients with DVT.
Huntington's disease	A neuro-degenerative genetic disease resulting in unsteady gait, lack of coordination, and eventually uncontrolled movements such as chorea.	First detailed description of the disease among families was noted by George Huntington in 1872.

Wernicke aphasia	It is a sensory aphasia, or receptive aphasia, where the patients are unable to process the information they receive, either through written or spoken language.	This aphasia is named after German physician Carl Wernicke who located the sensory area for language comprehension in the brain.
Whipple's procedure	This is a procedure conducted to treat tumors or disorders of the pancreas, bile duct, and intestine. Portions of the head of the pancreas, duodenum, bile duct, and gallbladder are removed.	Allen Oldfather Whipple refined the complex pancreatico-duodenectomy, reducing it to a one-step procedure. He is also known for Whipple's triad used to identify insulinomas.

Medical Acronyms

A lot of multi-word medical terms are commonly written as acronyms or abbreviated forms based on the first letters of each word. This will occur in medical texts and journal articles, as well as routine medical documents.

Acronyms are frequently formed using the capitalized first letters of the full medical term. This is not a strict rule, since some acronyms can be in lowercase or are formed by capitalizing lowercase letters within a word, such as ECG for electrocardiogram.

Listen to track 20

Acronym	Medical Term
ABC	Airway Breathing Circulation
ABG	Arterial Blood Gas
ACE(I)	Angiotensin Converting Enzyme (Inhibitor)
ADHD	Attention Deficit Hyperactivity Disorder
AF	Atrial Fibrillation
AIDS	Acquired Immunodeficiency Syndrome
ARDS	Acute Respiratory Distress Syndrome
BMI	Body Mass Index
BPH	Benign Prostatic Hyperplasia
CABG	Coronary Artery Bypass Graft
CAT/CT scan	Computed Axial Tomography
CHF	Congestive Heart Failure
COPD	Chronic Obstructive Pulmonary Disease
CSF	Cerebrospinal Fluid
CVA	Cerebrovascular Accident
CXR	Chest X-ray
DM	Diabetes Mellitus
DNR	Do Not Resuscitate
DVT	Deep Vein Thrombosis
ECG	Electrocardiogram
ECT	Electroconvulsive Therapy
EEG	Electroencephalogram
ET	Endotracheal Tube
FB	Foreign Body
FHR	Fetal Heart Rate
FX	Fracture

Chapter 6: Using Medical Homonyms, Eponyms, Acronyms, Abbreviations, and Symbols

GERD	Gastroesophageal Reflux Disorder
GFR	Glomerular Filtration Rate
GI	Gastrointestinal
GU	Genitourinary
HR	Heart Rate
HRT	Hormone Replacement Therapy
HTN	Hypertension
IBD	Inflammatory Bowel Disease
IBS	Irritable Bowel Syndrome
ICU	Intensive Care Unit
IUD	Intrauterine Device
KVO	Keep Vein Open
MRI	Magnetic Resonance Imaging
MS	Multiple Sclerosis
MVA	Motor Vehicle Accident
NG	Nasogastric
NSAID	Non-Steroidal Anti-Inflammatory Drug
OCD	Obsessive Compulsive Disorder
PEA	Pulseless Electrical Activity
PID	Pelvic Inflammatory Disorder
PPIs	Proton Pump Inhibitors
PT	Prothrombin Time
PTT	Partial Thromboplastin Time
SAH	Subarachnoid Hemorrhage
SLE	Systemic Lupus Erythematosus
STD	Sexually Transmitted Disease
SZ	Seizure
TAH	Total Abdominal Hysterectomy
THR	Total Hip Replacement

TKR	Total Knee Replacement
UA	Urine Analysis
URI	Upper Respiratory Tract Infection
UTI	Urinary Tract Infection
V/Q scan	Ventilation and Perfusion Scan
VF	Ventricular Fibrillation
VTach/VT	Ventricular Tachycardia

Medical Abbreviations

Similar to the medical acronyms we just looked at, medical abbreviations are used to shorten often long medical terms or phrases. Medical abbreviations save time when writing out long medical terms and are also standardized so that everyone within a medical team can understand what specific abbreviation indicates.

Abbreviation	Meaning
Abbreviations used in medical pharmacology	
a.c.	to be taken before meals
p.c.	to be taken after meals
b.i.d.	to be taken twice daily
cap	capsule
gtt	drops
IM	route of administration is intramuscular
K	potassium
KCL	potassium chloride
Na	sodium

O.D.	right eye
O.S.	left eye
O.U.	both eyes
PR	per rectum
qd	to be taken daily
qid	to be taken four times a day
qod	to be taken every other day
qh	every hour
q2h	every two hours
q3h	every three hours
qAM	to be taken every morning
qPM	to be taken every evening
qhs	taken every night around bedtime
STAT	given or conducted immediately
Abbreviations used in surgery or treatment	
BKA	Below the Knee Amputation
in vivo	in the body
in vitro	outside the body, in an artificial environment (e.g. a test tube)
LLQ	Left Lower Quadrant
LUQ	Left Upper Quadrant
RLQ	Right Lower Quadrant
RUQ	Right Upper Quadrant
tab	tablet

Abbreviations used for assessment, diagnostics and documentation	
a/g	albumin to globulin
BP	Blood Pressure
C&S	Culture and Sensitivity test
CC	Chief Complaint
CBC	Complete Blood Count
D/C	to be discontinued
DC	to be discharged
DOE	Dyspnea On Exertion
DTR	Deep Tendon Reflexes
dx	diagnosis
LBP	Lower Back Pain
N/V	Nausea and Vomiting
PCO2	Partial Pressure of Carbon Dioxide
PO2	Partial Pressure of Oxygen
T	Temperature

Medical Symbols

Symbols in the medical terminology perform similar functions to those of acronyms and abbreviations. They help to shorten documented communication and since they are standardized, symbols are understood by everyone working in a healthcare setting. Symbols are used for measurements, indicating drug names, or expressing quantity.

Chapter 6: Using Medical Homonyms, Eponyms, Acronyms, Abbreviations, and Symbols

Symbol	Definition
≈	approximately
α	symbol used for alpha-adrenergic blockers
@	at
ã	before
Δ	to change
1o, 2o, 3o	indicating first, second or third degrees
↑	increase
↓	decrease
♀	female
♂	male
<	less than
>	greater than
=	equal to
∅	Null
μ	micro
+ / +ve	positive
- / -ve	negative

Chapter Recap

Medical homonyms are medical terms that have similar pronunciation but differ in spellings and their meaning. In common medical conversations, it is relatively easy to get confused if you are unaware of the meaning of the medical terms along with their designated spellings.

Eponyms in medicine are often inspired by the person who either invented a medical procedure, discovered a body part or documented a specific disease process. There is a long list of eponyms among medical terms.

Medical acronyms and abbreviations are shortened forms of frequently used medical terms. Since they are standardized they can be seamlessly used within medical documentation as well, to limit the time taken especially for writing out long and complex medical terms.

Medical symbols are used to designate certain measurements and quantities or to indicate certain features of drugs or conditions.

Chapter 6: Using Medical Homonyms, Eponyms, Acronyms, Abbreviations, and Symbols

Practice Exercise

Select the correct option for the following:

1. What does the following word mean: Enuresis
   - (A) Fecal incontinence
   - (B) Inability to pass urine
   - (C) Urinary incontinence
   - (D) Weak bladder

2. Select the correct acronym for Computed Axial Tomography
   - (A) CT
   - (B) CRT
   - (C) CXR
   - (D) CXT

3. What does the abbreviation "qhs" mean?
   - (A) around bedtime
   - (B) every evening
   - (C) every morning
   - (D) twice a day

4. What is the abbreviation for the right eye?
   - (A) O.D.
   - (B) O.E.
   - (C) O.S.
   - (D) O.U.

5. Which symbol means "to change"?
   - (A) Δ
   - (B) ≈
   - (C) ø
   - (D) ∞

Refer to Chapter 11 for the answers.

Chapter 7: How to Pluralize Medical Terms

For pluralizing medical words there are a few general rules. Understanding these rules is essential since many medical terms are derived from Latin and Greek, and the simple rules for pluralizing English words don't always work.

In this chapter, we will look into the most common rules for pluralizing medical terms. Be sure to watch out for exceptions to these general pluralizing rules as well.

Listen to track 21

Rule for pluralization	Example
For medical terms ending in **-a** the plural is formed by adding **-e**.	ven**a** = ven**ae**
For medical terms ending with **-ex/-ix** the plural form is made by adding **-ices**.	ap**ex** = ap**ices** append**ix** = append**ices**
For medical terms ending in **-nx** the plural is formed by removing the -x and adding **-ges**.	phala**nx** = phalan**ges**
If a medical term ends in **-x** then a plural is formed by adding **-ces**.	thora**x** = thora**ces**
Some medical terms ending in **-is** are pluralized by replacing the -i with **-e**.	test**is** = test**es** *Exceptions:* epididymis = epididymides femoris = femora iris = irides

For some medical terms ending in **-on** the plural is formed by replacing it with **-a**.	gangli**on** = gangli**a**
A similar rule applies for medical terms ending in **-um** where a plural is formed by replacing -um with **-a**.	osti**um** = osti**a**
For medical words ending in **-us**, it is replaced with an **-i**.	ram**us** = ram**i** **Exceptions:** corpus = corpora plexus = plexuses viscus - viscera
If a medical term ends in the suffix **-itis** a plural is formed by adding **-itides**.	arthr**itis** = arthr**itides**
For medical terms ending with **-y** the plural is formed by adding **-ies**.	cavi**ty** = cavi**ties**
In words ending with **-yx**, the x is replaced with a **-ces**.	caly**x** = caly**ces**
Medical terms ending with **-oma/-ma** are pluralized by adding **-ta**.	sto**ma** = stoma**ta**
For some medical words the singular and plural forms are the same.	meatus = meatus

For medical terms made up with two words, their plurals are formed through pluralizing both the words, especially for medical terms derived from Latin.	ven**a** cav**a** - ven**ae** cav**ae**
A few words do not follow the general rules of medical pluralization.	cornu = cornu**a** vas = vas**a** pons = pon**tes**

Many medical terms have direct English meanings. This means pluralizing them will follow a similar pattern as observed in the English language. The following are a few examples of these rules.

Listen to track 22

Most English words can be pluralized by adding an **-s** to the end of the word.	finger = finger**s**
English words ending in **-s** are pluralized by adding **-es**.	recess = recess**es**
English medical words ending in **-ch/-x/-sh** are also pluralized by adding **-es**.	stit**ch** = stitch**es** flex = flex**es** cru**sh** = crush**es**
Medical words ending with a **consonant followed by a -y** are pluralized by replacing the y with **-ies**.	neuropathy = neuropath**ies**

Medical words ending with a consonant followed by an -**o** are pluralized by adding -**nes**.	comed**o** = comedo**nes** *Exceptions:* embryo = embryos placebo = placebos

There are a few rules for pluralizing abbreviations and acronyms.

Abbreviations used to denote measurements are recorded without pluralization if there is a fixed value.	Her cervix is 4 **cm** dilated. (Not 4 cms.)
Single digits are pluralized with an -**'s**.	He counted his steps in 5**'s**.
Double-digit numbers are pluralized by adding an -**s**.	He was in his 30**s**.
Acronyms in upper case are pluralized by adding an -**s**.	RBC**s**
Lowercase acronyms are pluralized with an -**'s**.	wbc**'s**

Chapter Recap

Since many medical words are derived from either Latin or Greek they do not follow the general rules for pluralization. For the comprehension of medical terms, especially within medical texts, understanding how plurals are formed is essential. Understanding the simple rules of pluralization also helps with documentation. A few medical words have direct English meanings. These medical terms frequently follow the standard rules of pluralization in the English language.

Practice Exercise

Select the correct plural form:

1. Apex
   (A) Apexes
   (B) Apexs
   (C) Apices
   (D) Apeces

2. Femoris
   (A) Femora
   (B) Femores
   (C) Femorises
   (D) Femori

3. Sarcoma
   (A) Sarcomas
   (B) Sarcomata
   (C) Sarcome
   (D) Sarcomices

4. Placenta previa
   (A) Placenta previae
   (B) Placentae previa
   (C) Placentae previae
   (D) Placentas previas

5. Cornu
   (A) Corni
   (B) Cornu
   (C) Cornua
   (D) Cornui

Refer to Chapter 11 for the answers.

Chapter 8: Understanding the Structure and Organization of the Body

For easier reference to particular sections of the body, especially during medical imaging and documentation, the body is divided into specific regions.

The region-specific medical terms are first documented during physical examination where changes in appearance or marks are recorded. This helps imaging technicians to understand the best location or position to conduct a test in order to get the best view of the affected organ.

The lines used to organize the body into sections are, of course, imaginary. However, these divisions are standardized in their usage across medical fields. This makes for easier communication and fewer misunderstandings.

In this chapter, we will look through the various terms used when describing the structure and organization of the body.

Medical Terms for Anatomical Planes

Anatomical planes are imaginary parallel and perpendicular lines dividing the body into four specific sections.

Listen to track 23

Anatomical Plane	Description
Coronal	Also known as the frontal plane, the coronal plane divides the body into anterior (front) and posterior (back) sections.

Transverse	This is a plane parallel to the ground, marked through the waistline. It divides the body into upper and lower sections.
Sagittal/Midsagittal	This type of sagittal plane is drawn exactly in the body's midline, sectioning it into right and left portions.
Parasagittal	This vertical plane divides the body into left and right sections.

Medical Terms for Anatomical Body Positions

While carrying out a patient's physical examination or during certain clinical procedures, positioning a patient for accurate organ access becomes important. During a physical exam if patient is either standing, sitting, or lying down in a specific position this could assist with examining certain organ systems better to provide more accurate results.

The following table lists a few of the most common medical terms for positions patients are placed in during clinical exams and procedures.

Listen to track 24

Anatomical Body Position	Description
Erect	Standing upright
Supine	Lying down on one's back, also known as dorsal recumbent.
Prone	Lying down with face and abdomen on the examination table.

Lateral Recumbent	Lying down on one side, either left or right.
Sims	Lying down on the left side, with the right thigh and knee, slightly pulled toward the chest.
Fowler	Semi-seated position, where the head is raised between a 45- 60° angle, and the patient's legs are either bent or straight.
Lithotomy	While the patient is lying supine, then the thighs are moved apart and the legs are either drawn to the abdomen or supported in stirrups.
Trendelenburg	While the patient is supine, the head of the bed is lowered to a 15-30° angle so that the legs are at an elevated position relative to the head.
Reverse Trendelenburg	While the patient is lying supine, the head and chest are elevated to a 30° angle, as the legs continue to remain in their position on the examination table.
Genupectoral	The knees and thighs are upright on the examination table, while the upper chest and face are lowered to the bed. This is also known as the knee-chest position.

Medical Terms for the Various Regions of the Body

Medical terms for regions of the body help to designate the specific organs or tissues present within that part of the body. This is especially useful when a patient presents with a specific medical complaint, either stating or pointing to the specific region of their body.

Body regions are standardized within medical text and documentation. Knowing the various body regions can assist you as a physician in effectively ruling in (and also ruling out) possible underlying causes for the patient's concerns.

Abdominal Regions

The abdomen is broadly classified into four quadrants.

Abdominal quadrant	Underlying organs
RUQ Right Upper Quadrant	Liver
	Gallbladder and biliary tree
	Head of pancreas
	Duodenum
	Right kidney
	Hepatic flexure of large intestine
LUQ Left Upper Quadrant	Stomach
	Spleen
	Pancreas
	Left liver lobe
	Splenic flexure and a portion of the transverse colon
	Left kidney

RLQ Right Lower Quadrant	Appendix Right ureter Cecum and ascending colon Right ovary and fallopian tube in females
LLQ Left Lower Quadrant	Left ureter Descending and sigmoid colon Left ovary and fallopian tube in females

The abdomen is then further subdivided into nine specific regions.

Listen to track 25

Abdominal region	Location on abdomen	Underlying organs
Right hypochondriac	Located below the right side of the ribcage.	Gallbladder Right lobe of liver Ascending and transverse colon Portion of the small intestine Right kidney

Epigastric	As the name implies it is the area just above the stomach, between the hypochondriac regions.	Right and left lobe of liver Esophagus Most of the stomach Pancreas Spleen Duodenum Transverse colon Portions of both the kidneys Both the ureters
Left hypochondriac	Located below the left side of the ribcage.	Stomach Left lobe of liver Left kidney Spleen Tail of pancreas Portion of the small intestine Transverse and descending colon
Right lumbar	Found below the right hypochondriac region on the right flank of the abdomen.	Tip of the liver Gallbladder Right kidney Portion of the small intestine Ascending colon

Umbilical	Area located around the navel between the two flanks of the abdomen.	Stomach Pancreas Medial aspects of the kidney Both the ureters Transverse colon Portion of the small intestine
Left lumbar	Found below the left hypochondriac region on the left flank of the abdomen.	Portion of the small intestine Descending colon A small segment of the left kidney
Right iliac/ inguinal	Located around the right iliac crest beneath the right flank.	Appendix Portion of the small intestine Cecum Ascending colon Right ovary and fallopian tube in females

Hypogastric/ Pubic	Lowest part of the abdomen, located around the pubic bones.	Portion of the small intestine Sigmoid colon Rectum Urinary bladder Both the ureters Uterus and both the fallopian tubes in females Prostate and ductus deferens in males
Left iliac/ inguinal	Located around the left iliac crest beneath the left flank.	Portion of the small intestine Descending colon Sigmoid colon Left ovary and fallopian tube in females

Regions of the Spinal Column

Listen to track 26

Spinal Region	Designation	Description
Cervical	C 1-7	The cervical region extends the length of the seven cervical vertebrae in the neck.

Thoracic	T 1-12	Encloses the region of the rib cage. It extends the length of the 12 thoracic vertebrae. Each vertebra has its own set of ribs.
Lumbar	L 1-5	Consists of 5 lumbar vertebrae, which are the largest of all the vertebrae within the spinal column. The region is designated between the ribs and hips.
Sacral	S 1-5	Consists of five fused bones, referred to as the sacrum. It fuses with the bones of the pelvis forming the pelvic girdle.
Coccygeal	Co 1-4	The coccygeal bones, also referred to as the tailbone, are fused forming the end of the spinal column.

Smaller Regions of the Body

Listen to track 27

Region	Description
Auricular	area including and surrounding the ears
Axillary	region of the armpits
Buccal	interior parts of the cheeks located inside the mouth
Clavicular	marked on either side by the clavicles located above the breasts
Infraorbital	area beneath the eyes
Infrascapular	area in the back, located beneath the scapular bones on either side of the vertebrae
Interscapular	between the scapular bones
Mammary	area designated by the breasts overlying the pectoral muscles
Mental	region of the chin
Orbital	area encompassing the eyes
Pubic	area located beneath the pubic symphysis
Sternal	region over the sternal bone
Submental	below the chin
Supraclavicular	area above the clavicles

Medical Terms for the Body's Cavities

The body is anatomically divided into two main cavities, the dorsal (back) and ventral (front) cavities. These are then subdivided based on the area described in the body.

Listen to track 28

Body Cavity	Description
Ventral Body Cavities	
Thoracic cavity	Covers the chest region. Primary organs found are the esophagus, trachea, lungs, heart, and aorta.
Abdominal cavity	The central region, located between the sternum and pubic bones. The stomach, intestines, liver, kidneys, pancreas, spleen, gallbladder, and all linked structures are found within the abdominal cavity.
Pelvic cavity	Found below the abdomen, encompassed by the pelvic bones. The reproductive organs and urinary bladder are the primary organs present.
Dorsal Body Cavities	
Cranial cavity	The brain is the primary organ present within this cavity. It forms the superior region of the body.
Spinal cavity	Extends the length of the spinal column. It consists of the spinal cord and nerves that branch out from it.

Medical Terms That Indicate Specific Body Parts

Specific medical terms are used to indicate particular places on the body where a problem may exist. These medical terms are frequently used within medical texts and subsequently in medical documentation. Using these terms correctly prevents miscommunication, as describing an area of the body in ordinary terms can vary from one person to the next.

Listen to track 29

Body Part	Designation
Anterior Body Parts	
antebrachial	forearm
antecubital	anterior to the elbow
axillary	armpit
brachial	arm
carpal	wrist
celi(o)	abdomen
cephalic	head
cranial	cranium
crural	leg
facial	face
frontal	forehead
femoral	thigh
inguinal	groin
ocular	eye
oral	mouth
palmar	palm
patellar	knee

pedal	foot
phalangeal	fingers
pubic	pubis
tarsal	toes
thoracic	chest
umbilical	navel
Posterior Body Parts	
cervical	neck
gluteal	buttock
iliac	hip
lumbar	lower back
occipital	base of the skull
popliteal	behind the knee
sacral	sacrum
scapular	shoulder
tarsal	ankle
plantar	sole of the foot

Chapter Recap

Specific medical terms are used to describe the structure of the body and how it is organized.

Anatomical planes are imaginary divisions used to categorically divide the body into four viewing planes, namely coronal, transverse, sagittal, and parasagittal.

Medical terms for various body positions provide an idea of how a patient should be placed for relevant physical examination and various clinical procedures. These positions provide the best access to certain organ systems during a clinical exam.

Regions of the body in medical terminology are used to define specific parts of the body where particular organs or tissues might be found. This is especially useful for documentation and subsequently carrying out procedures such as medical imaging. The abdomen is broadly classified into four quadrants and further divided into nine regions. The spinal column has five regions. A few smaller regions in the body have specific medical terms to designate their location.

There are two primary body cavities, the ventral and the dorsal cavities. These are then further divided into five more cavities to assist with locating specific organs.

A few parts of the body have their own medical terms which help in identifying the specific location of an injury or problem.

Chapter 8: Understanding the Structure and Organization of the Body

Practice Exercise

Choose the correct option:

1. An imaginary vertical line separating the left and right parts of the body:
   (A) Coronal plane
   (B) Frontal plane
   (C) Sagittal plane
   (D) Transverse plane

2. The patient is made to lie down on his side with his right thigh and knee pulled toward his chest:
   (A) Genupectoral position
   (B) Lateral recumbent position
   (C) Fowler position
   (D) Sims position

3. The epigastric region is:
   (A) Above the stomach
   (B) Around the navel
   (C) Below the right side of the rib cage
   (D) The left flank

4. A region that consists of five massive vertebrae, making up the most flexible and supportive part of the spine is the:
   (A) Cervical region
   (B) Lumbar region
   (C) Sacral region
   (D) Thoracic region

5. Antebrachial is:
   (A) Arm
   (B) Armpit
   (C) Forearm
   (D) Wrist

Refer to Chapter 11 for the answers.

Chapter 9: Designating Root Words to Body Systems

In chapter 3, we had a comprehensive look at most of the root words used in medical terminology. We divided root words into two categories, namely, external and internal root words. This was based on whether the word is used to describe a surface body part or an internal one.

In this chapter, we will have a look at the root words based on the body systems they represent. These root words can then be used with various suffixes and prefixes to form medical terms that represent particular parts of the body.

Listen to track 30

Cardiovascular System		
Root Word	**Meaning**	**Example**
angi(o)-	blood vessel	**angio**ma: a small tumor of the blood vessel, frequently non-malignant
aort(o)-	aorta	**aorto**plasty: repair or reconstruction of the aorta
arter(o)/ arteri(o)-	arteries	**arterio**le: small blood vessels branching from an artery
ather(o)-	fatty substance	**athero**sclerosis: buildup of cholesterol, fats and other substances within the arteries resulting in the formation of a plaque

atri(o)-	pertaining to the atrium/atria	**atri**al fibrillation: an irregular heart rhythm originating and noticed prominently in the upper chambers of the heart, the atria
cardi(o)-	heart	endo**cardi**tis: inflammation of the inner lining of the heart
hemangi(o)-	blood vessels	**hemangi**oma: benign tumor of the blood vessels
pericardi(o)-	pericardium; protective sheath surrounding the heart	**pericard**itis: inflammation of the pericardial layer of the heart
phleb(o)-	veins	**phlebo**tomy: puncture made in the vein to gain access for either infusing fluids or drawing blood
thromb(o)-	blood clot	**thrombo**cytopenia: reduction in platelets diminishing the ability to form blood clots
vas(o)-	blood vessels	**vaso**constriction: narrowing of the blood vessels due to contraction of the outer muscular walls

Listen to track 31

Respiratory System		
Root Word	**Meaning**	**Example**
alveol(o)-	alveolus/ alveoli	**alveol**itis: inflammation of the small air sacs in the lungs, the alveoli
bronch(o)/ bronchi(o)-	bronchus/ bronchi	**bronch**itis: inflammation of the larger respiratory tubes within the lungs, the bronchi
capn(o)-	carbon dioxide	hyper**capn**ia: accumulation of carbon dioxide, observed by the increase in the partial pressure of carbon dioxide
epiglott(o)-	epiglottis	**epiglott**itis: inflammation of the epiglottis
laryng(o)-	larynx	**laryngo**scope: flexible tube used to visualize the internal structure of the larynx
mediastin(o)-	mediastinum	**mediasti**nal shift: occurs when one or more of the mediastinal organs moves out of its position
nas(o)	nose	**naso**gastric tube: a flexible tube passed through the nose into the stomach
ox(o)/oxi/ oxy-	oxygen	pulse **oxi**meter: device used to measure the blood oxygen saturation

Chapter 9: Designating Root Words to Body Systems

| pleur(o)- | pleura | **pleuro**dynia: following the infection and subsequent inflammation of the pleura, pain results in the area of the chest |

listen to track 32

Gastrointestinal System		
Root Word	Meaning	Example
append(o)/ appendic-	appendix	**append**icitis: inflammation of the appendix
bil(o)/bili-	bile/biliary tree	**bili**ary colic: pain caused due to the inflammation or passage of a stone through the biliary tree
cec(o)-	cecum	**cec**ectomy: partial or complete removal of the cecum
duoden(o)-	duodenum	**duodeno**stomy: a external opening made through a duodenal stump
esophag(o)-	esophagus	**esophag**eal varices: dilated veins located on the esophagus
gastr(o)-	stomach	epi**gastr**ic pain: discomfort or pain located around or above the area of the stomach
sial(o)-	saliva	**sialo**lithiasis: small stones formed within the salivary glands

Listen to track 33

Endocrine System		
Root Word	**Meaning**	**Example**
aden(o)-	gland	**aden**itis: inflammation of a gland
adren(o)/ adrenalo	adrenal gland	**adreno**megaly: abnormal enlargement of the adrenal glands
gluc(o)-	glucose	**gluc**agon: glucose regulating hormone secreted by the pancreas
glyc(o)-	glycogen; a storage form of glucose	**glyco**genolysis: metabolic process which breaks down glycogen to glucose
gonad(o)-	reproductive glands	**gonado**tropin: hormones released from the anterior pituitary that facilitates the function of the gonads
pancreat(o)-	pancreas	**pancreat**itis: inflammatory state of the pancreas
parathyroid(o)-	parathyroid gland	hyper**parathyroid**ism: excessive function of the parathyroid gland
thyr(o)-	thyroid gland	**thyro**toxicosis: state in which there is an elevated amount of circulating thyroid hormones

Listen to track 34

Integumentary System		
Root Word	**Meaning**	**Example**
adip(o)-	fat	**adipo**sis: an excessive accumulation of fat in a particular organ or all over the body
derm(o)/ dermat(o)-	skin	**derma**titis: medical condition or infection which results in the inflammation of the skin
hidr(o)-	sweat	hyper**hidr**osis: condition which results in excessive sweating
kerat(o)-	horny/ scaly tissue	**kerato**sis: skin lesion resulting in the excess production of scaly tissue
melan(o)-	dark/black	**melano**cyte: cell which releases the skin pigment melanin
myc(o)-	fungi	**myco**sis: fungal infection
onych(o)-	nail	**onycho**mycosis: fungal infection of the nails
seb(o)-	sebum/ sebaceous glands	**seb**orrhea: overactive sebaceous glands, resulting in excess sebum production
steat(o)-	fat	**steat**orrhea: excretion of fat in stool
trich(o)-	hair	**trich**otillomania: a mental health condition which results in the compulsive urge to pull out one's hair

Listen to track 35

_	Musculoskeletal System	_
Root Word	**Meaning**	**Example**
humer(o)-	humerus	**humero**scapular joint: articular joint between the humeral and scapular bone
ill(o)-	ilium	**ilio**femoral ligament: ligament joining the ilium and femur
ischi(o)-	ischium	**ischio**rectal abscess: an abscess formed between the rectum and the ischium
kyph(o)-	hump/bent	**kyph**osis: exaggerated curvature formed in the upper back resulting in hunched over back
lamin(o)-	lamina of the vertebrae	**lamin**ectomy: surgical procedure to remove the lamina of the vertebrae
leiomy(o)-	smooth muscle	**leiomyo**sarcoma: a rare malignancy which develops in the smooth muscle of an organ of the body
lumb(o)-	lumbar vertebrae	**lumb**ar lordosis: the inward curvature of the lumbar spine
maxill(o)-	upper jaw	**maxillo**facial surgery: reconstructive or elective surgery done on the face, upper jaw, and mouth

my(o)-	muscle	**myo**fascial pain: occurs due to chronic overuse and tear of certain muscles in the body
oste(o)-	bone	**osteo**porosis: condition where the bones become brittle and weak
scoli(o)-	twisted/bent	**scolio**sis: an exaggerated sideways curvature observed in the spine
spondyl(o)-	vertebrae	**spondylo**sis: degenerative changes of the spine, particularly arthritis of the spine
synov(o)-	joint capsule lined with the synovial membrane	teno**syno**vitis: inflammation of the synovial sheath lining the tendons

Listen to track 36

Nervous System		
Root Word	**Meaning**	**Example**
cerebell(o)-	cerebellum	**cerebell**ar ataxia: injury or disease of the cerebellum resulting in an incoordination of the muscle movement, affecting gait

Medical Terminology

cerebr(o)/ cerebri	cerebrum/ main portion of the brain	**cerebro**vascular accident: also known as a stroke, where there is a disruption in the flow of blood to the brain, limiting its function
crani(o)-	cranium/ head	**cranio**tomy: a surgical opening made in the skull to expose an area of the brain
mening(o)/ meningio	meninges	**mening**itis: inflammation and irritation of the meninges of the brain and spinal cord
neur(o)-/ neuri	nerves	**neur**algia: sharp, shooting pain affecting a particular area a nerve innervates, either due to infection or damage to the nerve

Listen to track 37

Sensory System		
Root Word	**Meaning**	**Example**
audi(o)-	hearing	**audio**logists: health specialists who manage conditions affecting hearing and balance
cochle(o)-	cochlea of the ear	**cochle**ctomy: either a partial or complete removal of the cochlea

Chapter 9: Designating Root Words to Body Systems

onjunctiv(o)-	conjunctiva	**conjunctiv**itis: inflammation of the conjunctiva often due to underlying infection
or(o)/ ore(o)-	pupil of the eye	**coreo**plasty: surgical procedure fixing the shape and size of the pupil
orne(o)-	cornea	**corne**al opacity: condition or injury that results in scarring of the cornea
ycl(o)-	ciliary body in the eye	**cyclo**tropia: a form of strabismus
lacry(o)-	tears	**dacryo**adenitis: inflammation of the lacrimal glands, ones that produce the tears
acrim(o)-	tears	**lacrim**al canaliculi: small channels within the eyelids that favor release of tears
scler(o)-	sclera	deep **scler**ectomy: a small opening is made in sclera to drain fluid, primarily to relieve pressure due to glaucoma

Listen to track 38

Urinary System		
Root Word	Meaning	Example
cyst(o)-	urinary bladder	**cyst**itis: inflammation to the urinary bladder

glomerul(o)-	glomerulus	**glomerulo**nephritis: inflammation of the glomerulus resulting from an underlying disease process
meat(o)-	urinary meatus	**meato**tomy: surgical opening made in the urethral meatus, especially when it is inflamed or enlarged
nephr(o)-	kidney	**nephro**pathy: deterioration in the function of the kidneys due to underlying disease
pyel(o)-	renal pelvis	**pyelo**nephritis: inflammation of the kidneys, primarily due to underlying bacterial infection
ren(o)-	kidney	**ren**al artery: arteries that supply blood to the kidneys
ureter(o)-	ureters	**uretero**stomy: external opening created in the ureter to divert the flow of urine
urethr(o)-	urethra	**urethr**itis: inflammation of the urethra

Listen to track 39

Female Reproductive System		
Root Word	**Meaning**	**Example**
cervic(o)-	cervix	**cervic**itis: inflammation of the cervix
colp(o)-	vagina	**colpo**scopy: medical procedure to visualize the internal aspects of the vagina and cervix
galact(o)-	milk	**galacto**cele: a cyst filled with milk found in the breast
gynec(o)-	female reproductive organs	**gynec**ology: the speciality of medicine which studies and examines the functions and diseases related to the female reproductive tract
hyster(o)-	uterus	**hyster**ectomy: the partial or complete removal of the uterus along with any supporting structures
lact(o)-	milk	**lact**ation: producing and releasing the milk from the mammary glands
oo-	egg	**oo**cyte: egg or ovum
oophor(o)-	ovaries	**oophor**ectomy: surgical removal of one or both of the ovaries
ovari(o)-	ovaries	**ovari**an torsion: when the ovary twists on its ligament and tissues

| perine(o)- | perineum | **perine**al tear: small tears that extend from the vagina into the perineum |
| vulv(o)- | vulva | **vulvo**dynia: pain in the vulva, frequently of an unknown origin |

Listen to track 40

Male Reproductive System		
Root Word	**Meaning**	**Example**
andr(o)-	male	**andr**ogen: a steroid hormone which facilitates the development of male characteristics
balan(o)-	glans penis	**balan**itis: inflammation of the head of the penis, the foreskin is unaffected
epididym(o)-	epididymis	**epididym**itis: inflammation of the epididymis, frequently due to an underlying infection
orch/ orchi(o)/ orchid(o)-	testes	**orchi**ectomy/ **orchid**ectomy: surgical procedure to remove one or both of the testes
prostat(o)-	prostate gland	**prostat**itis: inflammation of the prostate
sperm(o)/ spermat(o)-	sperm	oligo**sperm**ia: a low sperm count

Chapter Recap

Root words are the foundation of a basic understanding of medical terms. They are often linked with different prefixes and suffixes to describe various conditions, procedures, and medical specialties based on the part of the body involved. Specific root words are used for various body systems.

Practice Exercise

Choose the correct option:

1. Tiny calcifications in a vein: _____ liths
   - (A) arterio-
   - (B) hemangio-
   - (C) phlebo-
   - (D) thrombo-

2. Which of the following is not a root word of the urinary system?
   - (A) meato-
   - (B) pyelo-
   - (C) sialo-
   - (D) urethro-

3. Which of the following indicates an inflammation of the lacrimal glands?
   - (A) Dacryocystitis
   - (B) Conjunctivitis
   - (C) Cystitis
   - (D) Scleritis

4. A fungal infection of the hair shaft: _____ mycosis
   - (A) cochleo-
   - (B) kerato-
   - (C) onycho-
   - (D) tricho-

5. A benign tumor of the bone: _____ oma
   - (A) ather-
   - (B) lamin-
   - (C) my-
   - (D) oste-

Refer to Chapter 11 for the answers.

Chapter 10: Resources for Memorizing Medical Terms

We have looked through the basic rules for forming medical terms. But when it comes to memorizing these medical terms, there is no one-size-fits-all way to do so. For many of us, simply reading through a medical text can seem tedious without much opportunity to practice using medical terms.

Today, advances in technology have increased the options available at our fingertips for mastering medical terminology. Technology is making notes-taking, building mnemonic techniques, and even developing flashcards easier than ever.

Latest Medical Terminology Smartphone Apps

The world of medicine is continuously evolving. Technology has enabled quicker access to the latest information, as well as providing digital platforms to help expand our knowledge over time.

In this chapter, we will look through a few apps which focus on increasing your repertoire of medical terms.

Medscape

This is a universally known source for the latest information on anything medicine. This comprehensive application also provides expert commentary, drug and disease overviews, and importantly, activities to test your medical knowledge. A valuable feature is the search option which encourages the exploration of new words along with their meanings and images.

Oxford Medical Dictionary

This dictionary has over 12,000 entries, most of which are by healthcare professionals. Additionally, there are 14 illustrations and diagrams which help you associate specific medical terms with their respective body part or condition.

Dorland's Illustrated Medical Dictionary

Dorland's medical dictionary has over 40,000 medical terms along with their definitions and related illustrations. It constantly updates medical terms based on their current use and context. This app has been adapted from the medical dictionary that has been used for over a century by medical professionals around the world. An interesting feature is that if you are unsure of the spelling of a medical term, this dictionary suggests alternative words that likely will include the word you are looking for.

Med Term Scrabble

With over 30 word lists to choose from, Med Term Scrabble makes for a more interesting way to master the art of medical terminology. You can brush up on your knowledge in the form of the popular game Scrabble, but only through making medical words. This can also be a fun way to learn with peers as well as to improve your accuracy in spelling out medical terms.

Skyscape Medical Library

Skyscape is a comprehensive library on various medical topics. In addition to enhancing your grasp of various meanings of medical terms it also provides an anatomical atlas, as well as recommendations to diagnose and treat medical conditions.

This app is well known for assisting with pharmacological information as well as dosing.

Medical Terminology and Abbreviations

This app features tricky medical abbreviations and their definitions in medical terminology. Additionally, this app assists with using prefixes and suffixes to facilitate the formation of complex medical terms.

Taber's Medical Dictionary

This comprehensive medical dictionary features over 75,000 medical terms with 1,300 related images. A great feature within the app is the audio recording of difficult-to-pronounce medical terms. The app also hosts measurement guides, symbols, and videos.

Medical Dictionary – Healthcare Terminology

Most of the 180,000 medical terms present in this dictionary are supplemented with audio recordings of pronunciations, videos, and comprehensive explanations of diseases and definitions. You are also able to add your notes to this dictionary for future reference.

Learn Medical Terminology

A valuable feature of this app is the e-learning courses and interactive exercises. The app also hosts a comprehensive list of prefixes, roots, and suffixes. Using the search feature for new complex words can help you understand the formation of these words along with their definitions, making this a great facet of the app.

Flashcards

Creating medical flashcards is one of the simplest ways to master medical terminology. Each of us has our unique ways to learn new subjects. Flashcards become a valuable tool to assist with this process.

Flashcards are cheap to create and easy to use. You can create your flashcards in a simple manner that enables you to memorize medical terms. A few tips to keep in mind when creating your flashcards include:

- Avoiding too much information on each card. Keeping it short is an easy way to commit medical terms to memory.
- Group your flashcards into categories. As we have seen with root words, many of them can be arranged into their respective body systems. Consider unique grouping systems which will help you to remember the words easily.
- If possible, add pictures to your flashcards.

Flashcards are also available for purchase online or in medical bookstores. Often you can reach out to your seniors who may have their old flashcards, which you can make use of for your studies.

There are a few online applications that have preset flashcards.

StudyStack

This is a popular resource for flashcards, where students or teachers upload their flashcards. There is both an online web version and an app for StudyStack. Additionally, you can create your own flashcards, which can then be used to create quizzes to test your memory of medical terms.

Medical Terms Flashcards

These flashcards are preset to learn roots, prefixes, and suffixes. The app can also be preset to study mode, test mode, or memorize mode.

MCAT Flashcards – Kaplan National Practice Test

These flashcards for the MCAT (Medical College Admissions Test) include both printed flashcards and an accompanying app. There are over 1,000 flashcards that are categorized based on the subject areas, such as behavioral sciences and biochemistry.

Online Courses on Medical Terminology

There are several resources available online today to master the understanding of medical terminology. At the top of this list sits YouTube. Many medical professionals now take to this online platform to provide medical knowledge for free. Students can easily browse through channels that assist with learning medical terms. With ample choices available, the ones most tailored to your learning style can be followed.

Additionally, a few online programs facilitate the learning of medical terminology.

Des Moines University Free Medical Terminology Course

This free resource can be used by anyone who has a keen interest in medical terminology. The course is divided into lessons, with practice questions and exercises at the end of each one. Since the course is for everybody, explanations are kept simple, without the use of technical jargon.

Medical Courses and Certifications on Coursera

Several universities have uploaded medical terminology courses to Coursera. Based on your level of expertise, and the degree to which you need to understand medical terms, you can select a suitable course for your revision. Course durations range from one to six months. You can opt for various levels of certification based on the requirements of your profession.

Medical Terminology on edX

This course is provided by Doane University and is completely free. If you require a certificate at the end, a nominal fee is requested. Emphasis is placed on breaking down the medical terms into their prefixes, suffixes, and root words to provide learners with a basic comprehension of medical terms. In this course, an understanding of medical abbreviations is also provided, which is especially useful for those who will either encounter or need to write shorthand medical notes.

Medical Terminology on Udemy or Study.com

These platforms have several medical terminology courses available. Most of them require a nominal fee, but often they provide unlimited access to the course. Additionally, some courses provide certificates at the end if required for college credit. Not all courses are created through universities, so select a course based on your requirement for learning medical terminology.

Understanding Medical Words by the National Library of Medicine

This course is free and downloadable for offline use. Root words are broken down into Greek and Latin forms for better comprehension. Additionally, many of the terms have visualizations that help to learn their meaning. Finally, quizzes are also available to test your knowledge.

ExpertRating Medical Terminology Certification

This course explores medical terminology through an anatomical approach, dividing medical terms into categories based on the body systems they represent. Each medical term is associated with a practical usage case to enable a deeper understanding of the medical term. There are ten lessons, following which there is a final exam for receiving the medical terminology certification.

Guide Books and Workbooks for Reference

Guide books and workbooks summarize the most essential points required to memorize medical texts. These books are often available in your medical school library. They can also be purchased at bookstores or online.

These books highlight the important points within subjects to facilitate easier retention. For medical terminology a lot of these books can be used on the go, to practice both the pronunciation and application of medical terms.

Here is a list of a few guide books available for medical terminology:

- Medical Terminology: A Living Language
- Quick Medical Terminology: A Self-Teaching Guide
- Exploring Medical Language
- Medical Terminology: Easy Guide for Beginners

Chapter Recap

Mastering medical terminology can often require different approaches based on individual learning styles. While some can grasp medical terms through the simple overview of medical terminology text, others may need additional tools.

Technology has greatly expanded the number of tools available today for learning medical terms. Several medical apps, online courses, guidebooks and study aids such as flashcards have been developed to provide a comprehensive experience of learning medical terminology. Additionally, a lot of these resources provide exercises and practice quizzes to fine-tune your knowledge of medical terms. Finally, based on your style of study, using a combination of these resources might be the best approach to improving your repertoire of medical terms.

Chapter 11: Answers To In-Chapter Questions

Answers to practice exercise questions in chapter 2

1. Hypersplenism
2. Colectomy
3. Erythrocyte
4. Hepatitis
5. Tachycardia

Answers to practice exercise questions in chapter 3

1. Blepharoplasty
2. Pharmacodynamics
3. Hematoma
4. Xanthochromia
5. Osteomyelitis
6. Leukemia
7. Gastroenteritis

Answers to practice exercise questions in chapter 4

1. k
2. z
3. j
4. k
5. n
6. sk

Answers to practice exercise questions in chapter 5

1. Fusion of two surfaces
2. Half
3. Faulty
4. Procedure to gain access into a cavity
5. Within

Answers to practice exercise questions in chapter 6

1. Urinary incontinence
2. CT scan
3. around bedtime
4. O.D.
5. Δ

Answers to practice exercise questions in chapter 7
1. Apices
2. Femora
3. Sarcomata
4. Placentae previae
5. Cornua

Answers to practice exercise questions in chapter 8
1. Sagittal
2. Sims position
3. Above the stomach
4. Lumbar region
5. Forearm

Answers to practice exercise questions in chapter 9
1. phlebolith
2. sialo-
3. Dacryocystitis
4. trichomycosis
5. osteoma

Conclusion

Medical terminology is not only useful for physicians, but also medical coders, billers, administrators, and anyone working in the healthcare field can reap the benefits of a basic understanding of medical terms.

Hopefully, this book has provided you with the basis for forming and using medical terms for yourself. While it might seem like a lot to tackle at first, with regular use of spoken medical terms among peers, and continuous practice, you will be able to retain the rules and use medical terms effectively from memory.

While this book hosts simple quizzes for practice, consider using additional resources described in the last few chapters to supplement your study of medical terminology.

Thank you for choosing this book on your journey to mastering medical terminology. We hope you got a lot out of this book! We'd love to hear what you think. If you have comments, questions, or suggestions about this book, please let us know by sending us an email at support@medicfluent.com. This will help us to enhance our books and provide you with better learning resources.

Wishing you the best of luck with your studies, and all the new things you learn within the world of medicine.

Thank you,

MedicFluent Team

How to Download the Free Audio Files

The audio files need to be accessed online. No worries though—it's easy!

On your computer, smartphone, iPhone/iPad, or tablet simply go to this link:

https://medicfluent.com/medical-terminology

Be careful! If you are going to type the URL in your browser, please make sure to enter it completely and exactly. Otherwise, it will lead you to an incorrect web page.

You should be directed to a webpage where you can see the cover of your book.

Below the cover, you will find two "Click here to download the audio" buttons in blue and orange color.

Option 1 (via Google Drive): The blue one will take you to a Google Drive folder. It will allow you to listen to the audio files online or download them from there. Just "Right click" on the track and click "Download." You can also download all the tracks in one click—just look for the "Download all" option.

Option 2 (direct download): The orange button/backup link will allow you to directly download all the files (in .zip format) to your computer.

Note: This is a large file. Do not open it until your browser tells you that it has completed the download successfully (usually a few minutes on a broadband connection, but if your connection is slow it could take longer).

The .zip file will be found in your "Downloads" folder unless you have changed your settings. Extract the .zip file and you will now see all the audio tracks. Save them to your preferred folder or copy them to your other devices. Please play the audio files using a music/Mp3 application.

Did you have any problems downloading the audio? If you did, feel free to send an email to support@medicfluent.com. We'll do our best to assist you, but we would greatly appreciate it if you could thoroughly review the instructions first.

Thank you,

MedicFluent Team

About MedicFluent Team

MedicFluent.com has been created as a one-stop resource for medical professionals.

Whether you are pursuing the MCAT or looking to upgrade your knowledge of the latest medical information, MedicFluent aims to enhance your learning experience. Our website is continually updated with the latest in medicine. Along with guides within the website, we host a library of books from a variety of medical subjects to provide a tailored learning experience.

We understand that with busy schedules it can be difficult to review all the new information attained. This is why we have curated quizzes and practice exercises to sharpen your understanding of medicine.

MedicFluent is a free resource that can supplement your study of medicine. Our information is customized to enable learning in a fast-paced environment. MedicFluent can also be a reference guide for standard medical knowledge.

For additional information, please viit our website www.medicfluent.com or feel free to email us at support@medicfluent.com.

Short bio:
Dr. Michelle Frank
Michelle is a healthcare consultant and content creator with over six years of experience in the HealthTech space. She helped build three online women's health communities

focusing on judgment-free conversations for reaching practical health solutions. She contributes extensively to health forums, especially those centered on enabling wellness, advancing digital health, and FemTech solutions. She resides in India, exploring different cities and opportunities as they arise.

Your opinion counts!

If you enjoyed this book, please consider leaving a review on Amazon and help other language learners discover it.

Scan the QR code below:

Visit the link below:

https://geni.us/9bEwEM

Printed in Great Britain
by Amazon